1992

Managing
Health Professionals

Managing
Health Professionals

Michael J. Nelson

CHAPMAN & HALL

London · Glasgow · New York · Tokyo · Melbourne · Madras

Published by Chapman & Hall, 2–6 Boundary Row, London SE1 8HN

Chapman & Hall, 2–6 Boundary Row, London SE1 8HN, UK

Blackie Academic & Professional, Wester Cleddens Road, Bishopbriggs, Glasgow G64 2NZ, UK

Chapman & Hall, 29 West 35th Street, New York NY10001, USA

Chapman & Hall Japan, Thomson Publishing Japan, Hirakawacho Nemoto Building, 6F, 1-7-11 Hirakawa-cho, Chiyoda-ku, Tokyo 102, Japan

Chapman & Hall Australia, Thomas Nelson Australia, 102 Dodds Street, South Melbourne, Victoria 3205, Australia

Chapman & Hall India, R. Seshadri, 32 Second Main Road, CIT East, Madras 600 035, India

First edition 1989
Reprinted 1992

© 1989 Chapman & Hall

Typeset in 10/12 Palatino by Best-set Typesetter Ltd, Hong Kong
Printed in Great Britain by St Edmundsbury Press Ltd, Bury St Edmunds, Suffolk

ISBN 0 412 33350 3

A catalogue record for this book is available from the British Library

Contents

Introduction

The idea for this book grew out of a series of lectures which the author conducted as a contribution to the management and personnel management module of the Southampton University MSc Course in Rehabilitation Studies. It is, therefore, written particularly for those managing people in the health professions both in the public and private sectors. In many ways, health services are not different from any other service industry or, indeed, any manufacturing industry. The managing, organizing, motivating and general looking after people at work is universally recognized as the fundamental key to the performance of an organization. Unless an organization gets its 'people bit' right it fails.

The study of people at work has tended to become more complex over the years. This is partly because personnel management commentators and researchers have made it so, but mainly as a result of the increasing appreciation that people at work are complex organisms. They come to work for many different reasons; they have widely different abilities and ambitions; they have moods; they get ill, stale, out of date and yet can have great energy and enthusiasm. They are affected by and, in turn, influence society at large, the economy, their local community, the political scene and most important of all the organization they work in.

It is challenging to get some degree of cohesion and common purpose injected into people at work; at the same time making full use of their abilities and energy and by so doing fulfil the aims of the organization.

The complexities, problems and challenges of professional health staff management are such that books of this sort are warranted. Its aim is to describe the main personnel management elements in managing health professionals. Some are unique to such groups, some are more general. A further aim is to give some degree of knowledge and appreciation of such personnel management issues and techniques to help managers organize and motivate their staff better and so to improve the effectiveness and quality on the part of the organization for which they are responsible.

Until levels of senior management are reached, it is the norm for professional groups to be managed by and large by one of their own professions. However, with developments in management principles, this emphasis is changing to allow for more management to be undertaken by those trained as managers. Such a development will only pose a threat to those professionals who aspire to be managers but are only prepared to stick rigidly within the culture and constraints of their own original profession. Those who aspire to a wider managerial approach will make progress as long as they become competent in management, having previously demonstrated a competence in their own profession. Having done both, and gained respect in both, they will be able to manage any staff group whatever its origins.

The term 'health professions' can be a wide one. This book takes it to be those groups of staff in the health industry that provide diagnostic and therapeutic services and care to patients in the community or in institutions. Those staff groups, to justify being termed 'professional', need to have a body of general and specialist knowledge that is expertly used in the exercise of the profession, a system that defines and maintains policies, standards and conduct, and trains those working within it. In such matters, many professions regard themselves, often correctly, as largely self-managing. In matters of managing, planning and organizing work within a general health setting such as a hospital they are not. Groups and individuals need management of an extended and to some extent a different sort, that requires knowledge and skills learned usually, though not invariably, from outside the individual professions.

Health professionals face unique problems in that they work in an extremely multiprofessional setting. In a hospital there are no professions (with the possible exception of the Law) and few trades not represented. This complexity on its own puts the health professions in a different position than most others. More significant is the fact that the bulk of the work of the non-medical professions is directed or determined by a group (doctors) which works within the organization and is employed by it, but only to a limited extent is accountable to it.

This book is not intended to be a conglomeration of management experiences and facts. Nor does it try to be a textbook. It is more a discussion on the context of the processes involved in managing health professionals with comment and analysis on particularly important features, knowledge and skills involved in management of people doing the professional clinical work. The aim is that managers will become clearer as to their roles and tasks, and more aware of the tools available to help them, as well as the constraints that exist. This understanding will help them to manage complex organizations better with more benefit accruing to the customers.

Most of the book is written from a personnel manager's perspective but it is clear that if a manager of any sort is not adept at personnel management he can never succeed in the wider role and by reading and being influenced by it managers, in the health services especially, will gain some new insights into management and some ideas, knowledge and skills that they can put to good use.

The male pronoun is generally used in this book. The only reason for this is ease of reading and does not imply in any way that managers or other staff either inside or outside health services are or should be male.

Part One

The Personnel
Management Brief

Chapter 1

The management
and personnel functions

Whenever one or more people use their skills for the benefit of
an organization in return for a wage, they need to be managed.
A self-evident truth perhaps but it is one that is frequently forgotten particularly in organizations that are largely made up
of employees who assume they are motivated or controlled by
some professional ethic. Also frequently forgotten is the need
for the organization as a whole to be managed; that is, planned,
organized, ordered, resourced, checked and reviewed.

GETTING INTO HEALTH SERVICE MANAGEMENT

Management is a process that many aspire to for various reasons. Some like the power or authority it brings, others are attracted to the status that comes with the word 'manager' in their
job title. Some are very taken with the process itself, they may
partly see it as a chess game in which they move the pieces to
a plan, reacting to moves from across the board, in order to
achieve the aims of the organization – in short to win. However, many fall almost by accident into management and this
occurs especially in the health services in the UK and even more
particularly in the groups of staff often referred to as the professions allied to medicine. Very often in the past, but still too
frequently now, skilled and time-served basic-grade physiotherapists or staff nurses are appointed to more senior posts with
little prediction of their supervisory or managerial potential
and usually on the assumption that because they have been
expert at their basic trade they will somehow be good at organizing and managing those in the same business.

Whilst a number of clinical professionals decide quite consciously not to develop their careers in to management but
rather to stay at the bedside or continue diagnosing and treat-
ing patients for the bulk of their time, large numbers decide
they should develop managerially for reasons already men-
tioned. Often, however, it is because that is the only way in
which they can progress in their career, especially in promo-
tional and financial terms. In the health industry only medical
and dental staff can reach what is seen as the top of their profession and still spend the vast majority of their time and skill
practising the trade and skills they first set out to learn when
joining their chosen profession. It is, of course, possible for
senior doctors and dentists to be promoted into purely administrative or managerial jobs but these are few; within the NHS
the figure is less than 1%.

In the professions allied to medicine, however, the story is
a very different one. The amount of patient contact and actual
practising of professional skills changes in nature significantly
with the first promotion from the basic qualified grade and
usually drops substantially with successive promotions. The
net result of this is that the more senior managers become the
more distance is put between them and the practice of their
profession or trade. This dilemma has been well recognized
by the professions allied to medicine for the last twenty years.
Various reports for most of the health professions have tried
to address this very issue. Most well known of these were the
Salmon and Briggs Reports on nursing [1], although the tenets
they put forward have now been overtaken by the philosophy
of general management propounded by Roy Griffiths in his report to the Secretary of State [2]. One result of the introduction
of the general management philosophy into the health services
is to encourage a professional from any discipline to aspire to
more senior management and in so doing assume managerial
authority over a number of different professional and trade
groups. It follows that the route for promotion is then a general
management one and not up a purely professional ladder. Any
discussion about management of health professionals must be
affected by, and take account of, the potential polarization of
managers from their original trade.

THE NATURE AND COMPONENTS
OF MANAGEMENT

Clearly such matters are partly for the respective professions to resolve. However, it is important to recognize the current practicalities and then try to improve performance for the benefit of first the organization and what it is in business for, secondly the individual practitioner and thirdly the profession. Given that the current practicalities are that management becomes a more consuming occupation as professionals climb the career ladder, an understanding of management itself becomes necessary. Almost all management tracts give some definition of management, some of which are succinct and useful, others not so. The tendency is that the more experience one has in matters of management the more blasé one becomes about being clear on the process or business in hand. Often, experienced interviewers will say 'I can tell a good candidate by intuition' or managers of long standing will comment 'I can manage by instinct'. All too frequently they are rationalizing the way they do things (often lazily) whereas what they should be doing to maintain their freshness is regularly to think about what they are doing, and why and how. This means that any manager should from time to time consider what management is. The two most important components, which are very much interrelated, are running the business and organizing the people. A manager at any level is concerned with both these elements but, almost invariably, the more senior a manager becomes, the more of his time is spent running the business. In particular, he will be most preoccupied with planning, setting aims, reviewing performance and progress throughout the business in a general way. The organizing people aspect of his job will still exist but will be more concerned with creating the right climate in which other managers can motivate staff and ensuring employees understand and are committed to plans, aims and what the organization is in business for.

The first-line supervisor, that is the manager who supervises basic-grade staff, will spend much of his time either doing the same sort, or slightly more skilled work, as the staff he supervises. He will also organize their work, their rotas, deal with their problems and motivate them. Very little management at this level is made up of work that involves a corporate, strategic or overall view but unless this first-line supervision is done expertly and consistently the business as a whole will falter. Even in organizations that have an apparently low level of supervisory control, for example where autonomous work groups have been developed and in commercial and public organizations where quality aids are used, there is a strong recognition that co-ordination of aims and work as well as motivation and leadership of staff remain crucial activities. There is little doubt that the first level of management is the foundation of any organization and it follows that it is more senior management's prime job to guide, direct and support the junior managers, having ensured the general direction of the business is valid, understood and has commitment.

The common themes in all levels of management are first those of organizing. Managers need to organize the resources at their disposal be they people, money, buildings or machinery, in the most economic and effective way.

Secondly, the manager must plan and be clear about what the organization, and his part of it, is in business for. In the health service, especially, this aspect causes managers at all levels many problems. In particular, a manager operating within a specific professional group may perceive a number of reasons for his existence not all of which may be consistent with each other. There may well be occasions when the aims of a profession are seen as totally at variance with those of a health authority. This difficulty will be explored in some depth in Chapter 7. Only when the manager is clear in these matters can he organize resources appropriately.

Thirdly, the manager must be an exploiter, not in the pejorative sense of the word, but more as the person who gets the best out of the resources available, especially the people. Such a process is clearly linked with the organizing role but more than this it needs to involve high quality motivation and leadership of the staff managed or supervised, to ensure staff give of their best in all aspects of their work. Increasingly this means staff being involved in, and contributing to, the planning of their services rather than having an overall plan imposed upon them and being told what to do. Such developments

presuppose that staff are well informed, led, trained and motivated to participate fully in the business in which they work.

Fourthly, all managers have the responsibility to implement
and comply with policies, procedures, regulations, what is
recognized as good practice, managerially and professionally,
agreements and the law. However, it is a recognized tenet of
good management that initiative and imagination need to be
fostered. Therefore, it becomes crucial that a manager strikes a
constructive balance between the constraints within which he
has to work and the need for encouraging and using new and
imaginative approaches to managing and working. In striking
such a balance it is important to draw a clear distinction between policies, procedures and regulations that really have to
be complied with and those that are stuck to out of inertia or
a felt need to have a passive support system which relies on
what are frequently constricting policies. In organizations where
a large number of policies or procedures exist there is also the
danger that policies can be cited to contradict other policies and
thereby militate against consistent action. All too often the un-
thinking manager when challenged on an issue by a member
of staff will respond that the employee should 'do it because
it is policy'. A manager who uses such a response more than
exceptionally could almost be replaced by a policy manual.

The importance of accountability

Finally the manager must be responsible for what gets done, or
not as the case may be, and be accountable to a more senior
manager or group in the organization. The notion of accountability is sometimes misconstrued. Many managers, for example, when allocated a budget will regard breaking even or
even underspending as the main aim and if they achieve that
they will expect their manager to infer that their job is done
well. Conversely, overspending is frequently seen as the main
management crime that needs to be avoided more than any
other. There are circumstances when budgetary considerations
may be paramount and it could never be argued that prodigal
practices are propitious managerially. However, budget considerations may not be paramount: budgets are a resource to enable certain things to be done and it may be that these things,

if they are what the organization is in business for, are superordinate. This being so, a manager who overspends in achieving
such superordinate goals may well be able to account, prospectively, contemporaneously or retrospectively for his actions.
If such an account is accepted the manager's responsibility
will have been discharged and whilst being held to account will
also be held to have been correct and proper. The public health
services in the UK are financed on the basis of cash limits. This,
in management terms, means that overall the books need to be
balanced or overspendings offset by underspendings, overspendings carried over into the following year or additional
funding sought for specific services.

The notion and implications of accountability are the key
to the way any organization does its work. It is also the key to
the sort of management hierarchy or structure that is created
to help make sure work is done and responsibilities are discharged in a timely and appropriate way, appropriate that is
to the aims of the business. The process of management has
not always been viewed in these ways: since the beginning
of the industrial revolution some two hundred years ago the
structuring and dynamics of business and service organizations
have changed frequently and often dramatically.

BUSINESS AND MANAGEMENT EVOLUTION

In the early stages of industrialization (although the concept is
applicable to earlier days) it became clear that the three essential
components of any business were land, capital and labour [3].
Land to build premises in which to make whatever the business
was set up to make; capital to provide funds to buy raw materials, build the premises and install machinery; and labour to
work the machinery to produce the goods. A fourth element
needs to be added, that of entrepreneurship or managerial flair.
This element was seen as the risk-taking owner who also did
the organizing. It was he who was largely responsible for the
'mill owner' reputation of many business owners and managers
who by and large regarded labour as a business commodity
just like land, machinery or raw materials and often seen as
less valuable and more expendable.

Through a fascinating history, the labour element tried to

redress this balance. Over a hundred and fifty years labour has been accorded more financial and moral status partly through the development of trade unions and the intervention of agencies such as government and industrial philanthropists. Whilst the actual balance changes over time it remains an economic and commercial necessity, especially in the manufacturing industries, for unit labour costs must be kept to a minimum. As the price of labour increases, alternative and cheaper factors of production will be used.

Development of the health services

Over a period a number of significant changes have taken place. The more important in the context of managing have been the increasing interest of and intervention by governments on behalf of society at large in the rules by which businesses are run. Initially, Parliament introduced laws that restricted certain practices to either; improve safety, keep certain groups out of the labour market, or protect various parts of industries, or to encourage others.

More significantly, in the twentieth century the public service sector burgeoned which not only created significant employment and altered the development of many skills and professions but also encouraged the development of the idea that service organized by the state is a worthwhile thing. The National Health Service [4] is the prime example of this.

A further change that has taken place is that the service sector has increased in size and remains labour-intensive both in cost and absolute terms. There are numerous reasons for such a change, the most notable of which are the changes in society which bring about an increased demand for personal services and that relatively little personal service work can be automated. This trend was particularly marked in the National Health Service from 1948 to the early 1980s so that now over 72% of NHS expenditure is taken up by the pay bill which supports more than one million employees.

New developments

These changes need to be seen in conjunction with the rapid developments in new and information technology. Many commentators see the introduction of computers, robotics and other forms of hi-tech technology as a revolution no less significant than the industrial revolution in the nineteenth century. The evidence [5] so far shows them to be right and managers at all levels and of all trades and professions need to recognize the new demands and opportunities that such a revolution brings. Not only do such developments bring material change but they affect skill mixes, attitudes, training, the need for different aptitudes and challenge the very need for certain trade and professional groups. Similarly, motivational techniques and the traditional nature of manager/subordinate relationships and hierarchical organization are brought into question. Examples of all these changes exist in the engineering industry, most extremely in that of Japanese motor manufacturing, whose methods are now being copied in most countries possessing volume motor manufacturing industry. In the service sector the impact of new technology in banking and other financial service organizations, for example building societies and insurance companies, has been phenomenal and highly visible in the high street. Retail services have also changed their ways of working, their size and their organizational structures markedly in the past twenty years, partly because of changing retail techniques as in supermarkets, but more recently because of the applicability of new technologies to the trade.

Specific developments in management and business techniques have accompanied these technological changes and their influence on work attitudes and society as a whole.

Such developments and the growing demands by employees for more involvement [6] in their employing organizations especially in matters that affect their working lives add weight to the view that managing any group of staff has become a complex process and though logic suggests one should simplify this, the reality is that complexities exist and at least need to be recognized and at best used to assist managing.

LINE AND STAFF MANAGEMENT

The fact that managing people and organizations has become so much more complex than it was fifty or even twenty years ago has led to the rapid development of staff management – as opposed to line management. More recently there are indications, especially in the health services where the evolution of general management and stronger beliefs in personal accountability have occurred, that the emphasis may swing back towards line management. We have seen that a line manager is one who is held responsible for achieving objectives or targets that are directly part of the business of the organization. The manager may well receive instructions from higher up 'the line' and in turn give instruction to subordinate staff and directly supervise their implementation. A foreman on a building site is a line manager as he directly supervises building labourers, bricklayers and so on. In the same way a senior physiotherapist or ward sister is a line manager in that they directly supervise or manage subordinate staff.

A staff manager is one who provides a support service to line managers at various levels. Such support might be expert specialist advice, provision of an administrative service, or of information and assistance with planning, training or other management processes. It may also involve certain elements of monitoring performance, for example a Finance Manager will report financial performance of particular managers to the General Manager or a Personnel Manager might report a labour turnover or the state of employee relations to the General Manager. Such processes are not forms of unilateral checking or internal espionage. They are much more to do with keeping senior levels of management in touch with the operational part of the organization and its health and then to help devise strategies and tactics for resolving problems and developing support systems and skills for managers at all levels of the organization. (Fig. 1.1.)

Staff managers' roles, however, must never be allowed to take over or confuse the responsiblilities of the line manager. It is the line manager who accounts for budgetary performance, who achieves business targets and who manages staff. The staff manager is only of use if he helps and supports in this without obscuring or confusing what should be a clear responsibility. It was Roy Griffiths who said it should be clear to anyone entering a hospital as to who is in charge [7].

In the context of managing employees, the line manager is also a people or personnel manager and amongst all the professional and technical skills that he and subordinate staff use

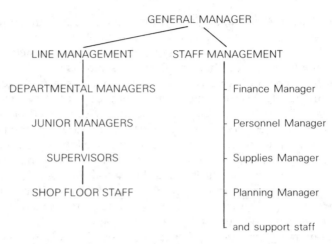

Figure 1.1 A typical organization of line and staff management.

in their basic jobs, he must exercise personnel management skills to an increasingly high standard. Whilst no staff Personnel Manager should ever suggest that the line manager is on his own if personnel advice is needed, the fundamental point is that the line manager is responsible for the result whether it be taking the rap for a mistake or credit for a success.

The staff manager has to account for his service both to his own manager and to the manager to whom advice or other support is being given. In a sense the personnel manager is more susceptible to market forces than most in that if the service provided is not relevant, expert, timely and useful, it will not be long before the service is not used.

Health professionals and personnel management

If the management of personnel is the province of all line managers, albeit with help and advice from a specialist, it follows that they need an increased amount of knowledge and skill in the subjects connected with personnel management, especially in the rapidly changing labour market. The acquisition of enough relevant personnel expertise implies a number of conditions: an understanding of what personnel knowledge and skill is pertinent to the particular management job in hand is one such condition. Much of this book is devoted to outlining such elements with a view to showing how they may be put to good use by most managers but especially by those who manage health professionals. This distinction is made not because health professionals are a race apart but because some of the problems and issues they face and the context in which they work have characteristics and a culture that are not common elsewhere in general employment, not even in other areas of the public service.

A second condition is that a health professional involved in management understands not only the general ethos and background to management and employment but has a deep appreciation of the culture and special complexities and issues involved in managing professionally qualified staff in delivering health care in a multidisciplinary setting.

A further condition is that the manager in this scenario is prepared and able to acknowledge that in the health services, professional groups cannot be autonomous and independent of each other and depend for their existence on the larger or-ganization, normally a health authority or hospital. In managing a group of professionals, the manager needs to appreciate that the aims of such a group may be in conflict with the aims of the larger organization or with other groups and that such a conflict is largely for the manager to reconcile hopefully to mu-tual benefit, but if not, with the balance of benefit falling to the larger organization.

The subjects covered by personnel management are best summed up by: any activity to do with people working in an organization. Although this is a fairly simplistic outline it sets the limits and implies the scale of the subject. The Institute of Personnel Management has outlined the scope and relative roles of personnel management succinctly:

> Personnel management is a responsibility of all those who manage people as well as being a description of the work of those who are specialists. It is that part of management which is concerned with people at work and with their relation-ships within an enterprise. It applies not only to industry and commerce but to all fields of employment.

Personnel management aims to achieve both efficiency and justice, neither of which can be pursued successfully without the other. It seeks to bring together and develop into an effective organization the men and women who make up an enterprise enabling each to make her own best contribution to its success both as an individual and as a member of a working group. It seeks to provide fair terms and conditions of employment and satisfying work for those employed [8].

People will naturally create new ideas and problems both individually and collectively that need to be tapped or resolved. Those people also have moods, peaks and troughs in performance, training needs, feel sick, do things incorrectly, can become argumentative and create conflict. They also bring to work values that they develop as members of a larger society and so will change their expectation of how they are prepared to be treated and how much they want to be involved in the business. They also expect to be rewarded in a number of ways for what they do; financially, with gratitude, with recognition of various sorts and with promotion. Collectively they need to be planned for, most of all in respect of how many types of staff and skill levels will be needed. Policies will need to be devised to make sure they can be recruited and/or trained and retained. Employers and employees also have to live and work within a political and economic climate and the law.

Despite the claims of many personnel management specialists, most personnel management functions and techniques have evolved as a response or reaction to the needs of employing organizations. In other words, such developments usually follow in an attempt to solve, rather than give rise to problems and issues in managing people. However, unless these responses are carefully considered and older functions or techniques reviewed or discarded, considerable conflicts can be created with the cure then potentially killing the patient.

The areas of personnel management that are of most use to those managing health professionals are discussed later in some detail. There are a number of personnel functions that are not debated at all or in any detail as they have only a very limited reference to the day-to-day practical management of health staff. Examples include the pay and conditions that are negotiated or decided at national level. This is a fascinating subject in its own right and one which many try to influence [9]. In practical terms most managers have to accept such things as they are and are well advised to spend their energy and expertise on those things they can effect.

THE PACE OF RECENT CHANGE

The outside observer of health service management would probably be most astounded by the sheer scale and pace of change in hospitals over the past twenty years. Up until the late 1960s, hospitals were administered in a way that was a cross between a paternalistic autocracy and amateurism – not always gifted. Typically, staff at different levels knew their place, got on with their job as was seen fit by tradition and were not, and did not really expect to be, consulted about changes, even those that directly affected them. This stability was to be disturbed by a number of changes, some of which have been touched on already. Further changes specifically in the field of personnel management need a little more discussion.

The growth of trade unionism in the health services

Trade unions in the industrial sense were non-existent in the NHS except at national level where negotiations on pay and conditions took place between civil servants and trade unionists who felt little need to change the ways they had worked for many years.

It was only with the advent of changes in the economy, political climate and society generally from about 1967–8 that a number of fundamental changes started to take place in health services trade unionism.

With a national pay policy it became impossible to negotiate levels of pay higher than inflation levels and yet some health service (and local authority) ancillary workers were recognized as being very low paid. The then Prices and Incomes Board in two reports [10] reconciled these apparently conflicting points by recommending such work groups could be subject to incentive bonus schemes. These are schemes where measured work done to a defined standard of performance is rewarded by payment of a bonus. The technicalities could be quite complex but the result was that staff at local level could now for the first time negotiate significant elements of pay because each incentive bonus scheme had to be jointly negotiated between local management and local staff. As a consequence for the first time there was something substantial (up to 33% increase in income) capable of negotiation locally. Such negotiations encouraged a well-informed and organized staff side and the ancillary unions which had up to that point been virtually dormant began to stir. They became well organized, canvassed for membership and generated expertise in both incentive bonus-scheme technicalities and negotiating skills. Union membership increased amongst the ancillary staff groups and with this came increased power and more negotiating success. It has to be said that most managements of the time were either reactionary or ill equipped to cope with such changes with the result that a fairly long period ensued in which many (often unnecessary) management concessions were made to the staff side. This naturally added an aura of success to the stirring unions which added impetus to the virtuous circle thus created. As a result, many more issues were seen as negotiable such as rotas, conditions of work, planned changes in the workplace and policies and procedure in all fields.

All the time national policy, society and the economy were moving and changes in attitude developing very rapidly to the point at which significant strike action became a reality in 1973 for the first time since the inception of the NHS in 1948. The issue was pay and in effect the staff won their case after sporadic nationwide industrial action by ancillary staff lasting six weeks. Because the trade unions and ancillary staff were so well organized and relatively expert and managements at national and local levels were not, the outcome of the 1973 dispute was almost assured at the outset. The significant point is that almost all the non-ancillary unions and professional associations then took a leaf out of the ancillary staff unions' book. They reorganized their structures, rewrote their rule books, changed their constitutions and began to show that if the ancillary unions could be proved right by might then they most certainly were prepared to climb aboard the bandwagon.

The net result is that now most staff and professional groups can be regarded as being organized, in the employee relations sense, into associations, professional or otherwise. Such associations are predominantly trade unions in the accepted and legal sense and are prepared and willing to act accordingly. Such a development, in less than fifteen years, has been a phenomenon unique to the health services in terms of its scale and degree and is a factor which every manager needs to recognize and take into account.

The labour market and health services

With the boom in the economy during the late 1960s and early 1970s the labour market became a much more difficult one in which to recruit. This applied to all groups of health staff, both trained and untrained, partly because there was a dramatic expansion in nursing and paramedical staff posts in the NHS in the 1970s and partly because relative rates of pay in most staff groups in the health sector dropped. Demand for adequate skilled labour has, since 1970, outstripped supply. Paramedical groups where this is especially so at present are occupational therapy and nursing. Other than in radiography and in pathology laboratories where technology is reversing the position, most of the professions are in a sellers' market. If implemented, Project 2000 – Counting the Cost [11] will exacerbate the situation in nursing by its proposed changes. Further stresses will be placed on trained staff over the next twenty years and the Project 2000 Report further highlights the already known and well-documented problem of the impending shortage of suitable 18-year-old girls (the traditional raw material for nursing) during the same period. By dint of thought, planning and action these problems, like any other human resource planning problem, can be overcome but it will take time, effort and imagination and some radical changes in the somewhat entrenched attitudes which predominate in some professions today.

Management restructuring of the NHS

As society changed considerable pressures were put on health services to adapt to changing demands. Since the early 1970s, consumers became more discerning and questioning about the service provided and their rights. Employees became more aware of their rights (and power to influence) and laws and regulations were increasingly introduced in the labour market generally and in the health services particularly to press certain policies or trends. Examples of this have been the move in 1974 to make the NHS more employee democratic. More recently, in 1984, there has been change from the almost exclusive use of traditional pay negotiating machinery to the development of a pay review body system bringing with it assumed independence and increased fairness. Perhaps most significantly, or at least most visibly, there was a recognition that the overall organization of the public health service was creaking. It took, however, three major reorganizations, starting in 1974, to bring the services' organization to where it is now. The current philosophy is based on the concept of a general manager [2] being identifiable and personally accountable for the performance of a region, district or unit with all the staff working in that unit being responsible to that general manager, albeit through a management hierarchy. Such radical changes over such a short period, with substantial changes coming before the previous ones have hardly had a chance to work or even settle down, have left their mark. A number of improvements are claimed to have been promoted which otherwise could not have taken place. It is clear, however, that a number of professions believe that general management is anathema to professional independence and strength as well as stultifying to career opportunity.

A relatively new feature of the current organization is the tight financial and planning constraints within which health services now work. In general, such constraints make for a good management climate in that problems have to be solved by thought and gaining genuine commitment rather than by throwing money at them and expecting this to be the all-embracing panacea. The planning constraint is more one of system or process and is linked to the need for economic stewardship of finances and other resources against the backcloth of increasing public demand for services and an ever increasing real need, particularly in the specialties providing services to the elderly. Managers of all services should with help; plan services against need, have commitment to financial policies and be skilled in financial management. In short, the manager of any health services staff now has to face most of the management problems and issues of any commercial manager with a few special ones thrown in. In addition, the health services manager has had to cope with a speed of development and change unknown in the commercial sector until recently in industries such as electronics or the financial and banking services.

Professional and managerial aspirations

Currently and for the foreseeable future, one of the main challenges facing any health services manager, remains not only being clear as to what the organization is primarily in business to do, but the fact that large groups of professionals see themselves needing to develop their profession often at the expense of the prime organization. Such aggrandizing aspirations do, and will, create tensions and conflict, not least because many clinicians and paramedical staff see management functions, for which they are prepared to be accountable to a general manager, as something completely separate from their professional functions. The two, of course, are interdependent. The management function is ultimately responsible for planning and organizing individual and groups of services to meet the overall aims of the organization. Services provided by professional groups must be planned and organized by – and consequently accountable to – a general and overall management function. The professional training or background of the general managers is irrelevant as long as they are respected, perform an overall managerial function and do not interfere with the day-to-day patient care work of individual professionals. The professionals' special contributions are to set standards, to police those standards properly, to maintain a unique body of skill and knowledge and ensure adequate training in these by ensuring the professions' field of activity is sensitive to changing needs.

The manager who manages health professionals also needs to recognize that professionalism can encourage, quite properly, individuality and that in a large organization, unordered individuality can lead to anarchy and an irrelevance to the main aims of the organization. Managers and professionals need to guard against too much standardization. To force uniformity can often stultify imagination and reduce initiative and energy. Non-conformity only becomes destructive when it is not channelled or directed and constructive dissent should never be seen as either professional or managerial disloyalty. Individual professional freedom is more to do with how a professional achieves success rather than the fields of work in which he or she operates. It is less to do with the what and mostly to do with the how.

By now it must seem that any health services manager has a gargantuan task. He has to become adept at management and personnel skills, to have a sensitivity to many complex issues and tensions that exist in any large organization. He must cope with very rapid rates of change, an apparently continually increasing workload and increasingly constrained resources. Furthermore, he is now held accountable in a much more personal way, which bears comparison with some of the more hire and fire commercial organizations. In addition, he has to work in a setting that is both charged with a great deal of human emotion (a direct consequence of the nature of its clients) and one that is complex because of the number of different professional groups which often have apparently conflicting aims with each other and their prime organization. Such a size of task is justified bearing in mind the importance of the product, the crucial contribution that staff must be encouraged to make and the fact that managers more than anyone else in the health services are stewards of public money. They have the right to expect support, advice and training in the various functions of management – most of all in the management of their staff.

REFERENCES

1. *The Salmon Report on Senior Nursing Staff Structure* (1966) HMSO, London; *The Briggs Report on Nursing* (1972) Cmnd. 5115. HMSO, London; Council for the Professions Supplementary to Medicine (1979) *PSM Education and Training. The Next Decade.* CPSM; *The Jay Report on Mental Handicap Nursing and Care* (1979) Cmnd. 7468. HMSO, London; British Association of Occupational Therapists (1981) *The Way Ahead*, BAOT.

2. *NHS Management Enquiry*. Letter to Secretary of State for Social Services from R. Griffiths (leader of enquiry) 1983. (Griffiths Report).
3. Smith, A. (1898) *An Inquiry into the Nature and Causes of the Wealth of Nations. 1776*. Routledge, London.
4. *The Beveridge Report on Social Insurance and Allied Services* (1942) Cmnd. 6404. HMSO, London.
5. Jenkins, C. and Sherman, B. (1979) *The Collapse of Work*, Eyre Methuen, London.
6. *The Bullock Report on Industrial Democracy* (1979) Cmnd. 6706. HMSO, London.
7. *Griffiths Report* (1983).
8. *Institute of Personnel Management Policy Document* (1963) I.P.M., London.
9. McCarthy, Lord (1976) *Making Whitley Work*, DHSS, London.
10. *National Board for Prices and Incomes Report on Pay and Conditions of Manual Workers in the National Health Service*. (1971) Cmnd. 4644. HMSO, London.
11. United Kingdom Central Council for Nursing, Midwifery and Health Visiting (1987) *Project 2000 – Counting the Cost*, Project paper 8, UKCC, London.

Chapter 2

Policies and constraints

During the past two decades it has been the stated aim of politicians, managers and administrators in all walks of life to roll back the frontiers of government and reduce the degree to which it interferes in everyday life, increase delegation and encourage initiative by increasing individual freedom. It is not germane here to analyse the degree to which such an aim has been achieved but it is necessary to comment on the fact that in most activities political, social, educational, in employment both commercial and professional, there is a strong predisposition especially in the public sector to bemoan the constraints both real and imagined that exist, to express concern about the constraining nature of policies and then when faced with a problem to express the need for a policy to cover it.

THE NEED FOR POLICIES

How often is heard the complaint on the one hand, 'give me the freedom to act in my own way and I will resolve the problem' and on the other, 'I have a problem and I think "they" should devise a policy to resolve it'? There seems to be a predilection amongst those managing health professionals, especially in matters of personnel management, to seek a policy to deal with what is often an operational issue. This is not always a bad thing; it may be that those propounding policy statements have not ensured those who need to know of them do so and how they should apply. There is no doubt that policies, especially in large employing organizations, are needed, are useful and save time. The unhealthy end of this spectrum is illustrated by the manager who, in effect seeks or demands a policy to resolve every staff management issue that ever occurs. In the extreme it is not difficult to envisage a management culture that has a policy statement on every such issue and all a manager has to do is to delve into the filing cabinet or switch on the micro computer, look up the problem and the policy that goes with it and then implement it. Such a way of working would create standardization but would totally stultify imagination, make no allowance for individual styles and, of course, not all circumstances can be predicted or squeezed into a mould.

Positive policies

Policies can be devised to ensure something happens. A significant example in the NHS has been the policy decision [1] to shift the emphasis from acute medicine to concentrate more on changing the way the mentally handicapped and mentally ill are cared for. Another example is the decision to accept the Griffiths Report [2] and institute a system of general management requiring personal accountability. It is easy to think of many local policies that are aimed at making sure changes take place, either in line with or to implement, wider or national policy, or to positively change some purely local circumstance. One of the most significant examples is the way all employers needed to authorize and implement local health and safety policies after the implementation of the Health and Safety at Work Act, 1974. Many personnel policies are designed to ensure something happens; a disciplinary policy or procedure will be designed to help managers act in a way that promotes fairness, consistency and ensures that those subjected to it are afforded all their rights in accordance with law or good practice.

Regulating policies

Policies may be designed to regulate what is going on in an organization. Many laws, especially those in the financial sphere, are predominantly designed to regulate the way in which things are done such as the Finance Acts, Companies Act, the National Health Service Act and most Statutory Instruments. Such regulation is aimed at promoting change or preventing a bad practice taking place. In the local employment setting policies designed to create equal opportunities monitoring, or planning and review systems are largely regulating, although they may stem from wider measures such as, for example the Sex Discrimination Acts. Such policies are not procedures. A procedure is the system or administrative mechanism that is set up to help the implementation of the policy. The policy is the statement of what is to be achieved by its publication.

Preventative policies

The third main purpose of a policy is to prevent something happening. To some extent prevention is the negative side of a policy that is designed to create change. The measures outlawing certain forms of discrimination are designed to promote equality and fairness. They are, however, often framed in a manner that is more preventative in that they explicitly state that discrimination is wrong and will be punished and only by implication encourage active moves towards equality. Some local policies can be perceived in this dual way. In particular many financial policies are seen as preventative or as constraints by managers who have to implement them, especially the policies that introduce savings or financial cuts or those that are to do with some of the more constraining financial standing orders.

GETTING POLICIES AND CONSTRAINTS INTO PERSPECTIVE

The reality is that laws, policies, procedures and systems are needed to promote necessary change, regulate behaviour and action and to prevent unacceptable or unwanted behaviour in society at large. The workplace in this context, as in so many ways, is a microcosm of society. Organizations of large numbers of people need structure and they need to know what and what not to do.

Custom and practice

It follows that managers need to know the constraints under which they work. Clearly many constraints exist as a direct result of policy statements such as the need for a defined level of expenditure. Many, however, do not. In the field of management, and especially in managing professional groups, a large number of practices and constraints exist that have evolved from the way things have been done. Such elements can exist through custom and practice and at times, because they are historically based, may well be inappropriate for present circumstances. Equally, many constraints are felt as apparent rather than real. It is often these that managers cite when suggesting that a particular change 'would be a jolly good thing and patients and staff may benefit but it's difficult because ' . . . 'it's always been done another way', . . . 'it's not consistent with policy', . . . 'we don't have the authority to change', . . . and so on.

Appearance or reality?

Such apparent constraints can outnumber the real ones in most employing organizations especially those in the public health sector. If improvements and progress are to be made a heavy responsibility rests with managers at all levels to question constantly the basis of any constraint or barrier to change and only accept it if it is real, substantial and in the overall interests of the organization. This does not imply anarchic or unilateral action, but instead questions the substance and reason for stated constraints. If they are apparent rather than real, then ignore them or change people's attitude towards them. If they are real, question them and plan open and legitimate ways of getting round them or changing them if the organization will benefit. Any healthy organization will have a culture and often a policy statement that encourages such questioning and will accept that neither internal policies nor constraints are immutable; indeed they should be seen as tools for performing the job that the organization is in business for. This means that the most important, in fact fundamental, policy that a manager at any level has to determine first of all is that which states what his part of the organization is set up to do. This needs to be in line with the higher levels but once determined it will help direct what other policies are necessary.

SOURCES OF POLICY AND THEIR
IMPLEMENTATION

There are several areas of policy that managers have to take into account and implement, but over which they have little influence.

First, there are the governmental, ministerial, Department of Health, regional and employing authority policies. Such policies cover almost every activity undertaken at local level and among the more significant are those to do with the management of personnel. Of these the most significant are the national agreements on pay and conditions [3]. The process by which change is brought about here is known to be tortuous and the outcomes are frequently criticized. Some groups try to find ways of interpreting or even circumventing the agreements that are made but generally they are accepted even though some might say there was little option in this for NHS staff. The private health sector in general uses the same pay rates and many of the conditions rather than set up its own pay-negotiating machinery so it can be assumed that the process brings some accepted order to a subject that affects all health workers. It is the responsibility of employing authorities and managers to implement national pay agreements and where some element of interpretation or discretion is allowed to exercise that in accord with the spirit of the agreement. Where discretion is used to interpret terms and conditions, either in an individual case or one involving a group of staff, the manager exercising discretion will need to account for his actions to his superior manager or, on occasion, to an auditor. The areas where most interpretation is possible are grades for jobs and starting salaries for new staff. On these, local consistency and fairness is needed as well as operation in line with the spirit of a national agreement.

The second group of externally decided policies which are important for those managing health professionals are those developed by the professional bodies either individually or collectively through the United Kingdom Central Council, the General Medical Council, the General Dental Council, the Council for Professions Allied to Medicine or ultimately by the Privy Council. Such policies are normally to do with training, education or standards of practice but others cover procedures for monitoring and ensuring standards, areas of demarcation between professions and certain disciplinary matters. Although these matters impinge on the managers' responsibilities and must, therefore, affect what he does and how he does it, the responsibility for ensuring that all its members are fully aware of them rests with the individual professional body. They do this continuously through the early pre-registration training and education and subsequently through post-registration training, communication and information, for example in professional journals and circulars. It is also incumbent on a member of any profession to keep themselves up to date and knowledgeable on all professional matters. It would be no defence to a professional misconduct allegation to claim ignorance of a professional policy or standard.

LABOUR LAW AS A POLICY AND CONSTRAINING FORCE

Labour law is a further external set of measures that has given line managers and personnel managers the most concern and problems for some years. Up to the early 1970s health managers felt they were very little affected by labour legislation. Not only was the NHS a crown body and explicitly excluded from much legislation but also there was a culture that suggested employment in the health professions was different from and loftier than most other forms of employment and professionals and, therefore, did not need to feel overly constrained by such prosaic matters as the law. The framing of labour law since around 1971–1975 has changed all this as has the general change in attitude in the health services, namely that health authorities are no different from any other employer and health workers are no different from any other workers either in the public or private sectors.

A higher standard for health services

The point has now been reached where there is reckoned to be no justification to treat staff differently on employment matters in the health trades than in any other employment setting. Some now might go even further and argue that the public health sector particularly should set higher standards of personnel management and be more positive in its compliance with the letter and spirit of the law than commercial concerns, merely because it is a public body. The fact remains, however, that many managers still have anxieties about how they apply labour law and codes of practice. Many feel constrained to be inactive especially in matters of enforcing standards and levels of performance and conduct through disciplinary measures because their perception of the law is that it has made it impossible to take any action with or against an employee because there may be some legal redress or some dire industrial relations consequence.

An understanding of the basic tenets of labour law is, therefore, essential for any manager if he is to have a clear idea of the constraints that govern the relationship between him and his staff, and the obligations each has to the other.

The employer/employee relationship

The fundamental relationship between an employee and employer is rooted in common law although much is now becoming enshrined in Acts of Parliament.

The notion that the employer is the master and that the employee is the servant still runs through significant elements of the relationship between the two. The employee, for example, may be expected to obey legitimate instructions and failure to do so may be reason to end the relationship. A legitimate instruction is one which does not in itself break a law and is a reasonable one in that it is both in the competence of the employee and within the general range of activity required or implied by the contract. Some of the more extreme notions that once lay behind the tenet of master and servant no longer exist such as an almost inferred ownership of the servant but the fundamental philosophy of principal and subordinate continues and is well recognized in law and in most employing organizations' hierarchies.

An area where statute law has subsumed much common law

is in the contract of employment [4]. Fundamentally a contract of employment is little different from many other contracts. It depends for its existence on an offer of employment being accepted and the intention and ability of both parties to perform their part of the bargain and to be bound by it. A contract is made once an offer of employment is made and accepted unless it is subject to express conditions such as a satisfactory medical examination. It can only be ended by either party giving proper notice, or by its fixed term (in the case of a fixed term contract) coming to an end or the job for which the contract was let being complete. It can also be ended by frustration which is an external event taking place, over which neither party has control nor could have foreseen, and which prevents the contractual obligations being met. Examples might be an employee being conscripted into the armed services or an Act of Parliament being brought in which precluded an employee from continued service by his present employer for, perhaps, reasons of nationality.

Most contracts end because the employee or employer gives notice for some reason. The amount of notice is laid down in either the statement of main terms of the contract or by statute (Employment Protection (Consolidation) Act, 1978). It is only legally fair for an employer to give notice of termination for one or more allowed reasons. These are laid down by the 1978 Act and are:

- a reason relating to the capability or qualifications of the employee for doing work of the sort he was employed to do. Capabilities mean skill, aptitude, health, physical or mental quality. Qualifications mean, amongst other things, a degree, technical or professional qualification relevant to the post held.
- a reason relating to conduct.
- a reason relating to redundancy.
- a reason which would involve the contravention of a restriction or duty imposed by or under a statute. The continued employment of employees required under statute to be professionally registered fall partially under this heading should they cease to be properly registered.

- some other substantial reason – which though it sounds something of a catch all, must be able to withstand the scrutiny of
  an Industrial Tribunal.

In the 1971 Industrial Relations Act, statute law created,
for the first time, the right not to be unfairly dismissed and
though that Act was repealed in 1974, its main principles including that to do with unfair dismissal were carried forward
in the Employment Protection Act, 1975 and the Employment
Protection (Consolidation) Act, 1978.

In the health services by far the most cases that reach
Industrial Tribunal are to do with capability or conduct of one
sort or another, usually exemplified by job performance, health
or behaviour whilst at work. The fact is that labour law, both
statutes and the body of case law that has resulted from it, have
made the subject of discipline and dismissal much clearer and
better understood than has ever before been the case. Added
to which we now have clear principles of fairness, equity and
reasonableness, together with a body of precedents to show
how those principles should be applied.

Labour law is now, of course, affected by the United Kingdom's membership of the European Community, in particular
in the fields of discrimination and trade union membership.
If UK law does not go as far as European law says it should or
if UK law is not consistent with European law, as ultimately
determined by the European Court of Justice, the UK Parliament is instructed to make appropriate amendments to its statutes. Individuals have the right, if they feel they have been
treated inconsistently with European Articles or Directives, to
take their case ultimately to the European Court of Justice and
a number have done so with success. Such success has subsequently brought about changes in the UK's legislation. Furthermore the Commission for the European Communities can
take a national government to the European Court, as it did
in 1982 when it was found that the UK's Equal Pay Act, 1970
did not comply with the equal pay for work of equal value pro-
visions of Article 119 of the Treaty of Rome. Following this
finding the government passed the Equal Pay (Amendment) Regulations in 1983 under which a number of women, including

some health professionals, most notably speech therapists, have taken or are in the process of taking cases.

The law and labour management generally

Statute law does not only intervene in matters to do with the contractual relationship between employer and employee. On average a significant labour statute is enacted every two years and although they do not have a unique bearing on managing health workers or professionals in particular they do show that intervention in the workplace by legal means is running at a high level.

Most significantly the law, other than its effect on the contractual relationship of employer and employee, has intervened in two main areas. The first is to do with what is generally called the employee relations fabric or machinery. Legislation has been passed to determine employees' rights in the matter of trade union membership and more recently non-membership, what trade unions may or may not do during and leading up to industrial action and to make clear the liability trade unions and their officers have for their actions. Such matters as these do not routinely affect the way in which a health service manager does his job; if a manager is faced with an issue to do with them, he would be well advised to seek expert advice.

Health and safety

The second area, in which the law has intervened affects all managers daily. It is to do with issues of health and safety. The turning point for most managers was the Health and Safety at Work Act, 1974. This Act for the first time, other than for specific work groups or work processes, brought the health services, and others, under a statutory obligation to have a mind to the health, safety and welfare of its employees, users and others. It laid down statutory duties and responsibilities on the employer, manufacturers and employees. Such responsibilities included the formulation of policies that clearly outline how health and safety issues will be handled, who will be responsible and what will happen in the event of failure. Also it made it clear that all local hazards must be identified and so far as is reasonably practicable the ways in which they be can made safe must be defined. Adequate training to enable systems of work to be operated safely must be given. The important issue on these matters is that responsibility rests where fault or lack of reasonable action lies. This means that almost invariably it is the local, operational manager who is responsible for the health of his staff at work and the safety of the systems of work that they use. Although senior management and employing authorities have certain overall responsibilities the local manager would be hard pressed to slough off local responsibilities.

Many managers attempt to pass the onus up the organization by suggesting that making safe an otherwise unsafe work system will cost new money. That may be so but the first responsibility of a budget-holding manager is to see if, by some adjustments, enough money can be eked out of the system to put the matter right even though output of work may in the short term decrease. The next move would be to bid for cash to make the required improvement. Senior management should, when granting the money or not, make some enquiry as to why the current system has become unsafe. The attitude of Factory Inspectors is clear: if a system is hazardous to health or safety it should be put right – otherwise an improvement notice or prohibition order will be issued. Ultimately they would take the view that if it was a choice between a profitable business being hazardous and a business going bankrupt through having to comply with safe work practices then the latter would be the course of action they would enforce – through the courts if necessary.

Failure to comply with the Act or develop safe systems may bring about action within the organization. It may also be that the Health and Safety Executive's Factory Inspectors will exercise their right to impose improvement notices which demand that improvements to safety are made. The Inspectorate may even impose a prohibition order that forbids a certain dangerous process of work being performed at all until specified improvements are made. Such sanctions can be, and are, applied to health premises. The Health and Safety at Work Act is not the only safety-related statute or regulation that applies to health work. It is, however, the widest ranging and can have an almost daily impact on a manager's work and serves to re-mind managers that the law is now a feature of most aspects of employment and staff management and needs to be taken into account in many management processes.

Vicarious liability

No résumé of labour law or constraints is complete especially for professional employees without explaining the principle of vicarious liability of the employer. To most it is apparent that should an employee commit a wrongful act which causes injury or damage to a third person, the employee may be personally liable. However, the employer may also have a liability that is vicarious. Clearly both the employees' and employers' respec-tive liabilities can only be adduced where the wrongful act has taken place in the course of the employee's employment. His-torically the reasons for the employer having a vicarious liability are twofold. First, as the master of the servant the employer has created the situation in which the employee has caused injury or harm – it is after all normally the health authority to which a patient has come for help. The second reason is much more practical in that, particularly in the health service, it is highly unlikely that the employee would be able to afford any major damages awarded. Often for this reason the courts hold the employer to be vicariously liable otherwise the plaintiff would not be able to recover damages in proportion to the injury suffered.

It is easy to imagine, as an example, a physiotherapist para-lysing a young sportsman by a bad or even negligent manipula-tion of the spine. The damages that could be claimed in such a case could run into hundreds of thousands of pounds. (1987 saw the first million-pound damages award in the United King-dom.) It is much more probable that the employer will be able to afford such damages. In practice it would also be highly un-likely for the employer to subsequently claim damages from the employee – if misconduct, poor or negligent performance were the cause of the damage or injury, the only practical re-course the employer has against the employee is a disciplinary one, which might of course lead to dismissal. In addition, the professional controlling body (e.g. UKCC or Council for the

Professions Allied to Medicine) might also discipline a professional and ultimately withdraw their registration that allows them to practise.

It is for these reasons that employing authorities do not require professional staff, other than medical and dental employees, to take out insurance. It follows, of course, that such employees, should they seek advice as to whether they should be insured against professional or clinical liability, can be told that such insurance has no virtue. The only valid reason for an employee taking out some form of insurance, be it through a trade union, professional organization or direct is so he may be indemnified against the costs of representation should he need it in an inquiry, court or disciplinary hearing.

POLICY AND CONSTRAINTS
IN THE INDIVIDUAL'S JOB

Probably the most immediate, continuous and important policy area for the operational manager is to do with determining the nature and detail of the job of employees under his control. It follows that a similar significance exists in the relationship he has with his own manager. It is not merely a question of outlining duties that need to be done, important though this is. The fundamental significance rests on the whole way the job, its nature and responsibilities are designed; how much authority is prescribed; how much discretion is given and how much the role is constrained. All too often little or no attention is given to the design of a job or the way in which it develops. With effective design not only does clarity ensue but the nature of the job itself can be used to motivate the individual and to actively encourage innovation and quality promotion.

In 1976, Rosemary Stewart [5] suggested there were three major components to any job. First the demands are what the employee cannot avoid doing – they constitute the core part of the job. Secondly the opportunities to organize some aspects of the job as the job holder chooses, she termed the choices; they would include not only how, when and where things are done but to a varying extent what is done as well. Thirdly there are the constraints – these are factors that put limits on what the job holder can or may do, such as policies, the law, regulations, custom and practice and the fact that time itself is limited.

Most managers [6], especially in the health services, seem to concentrate on the demands and constraints of a job when reviewing or designing it partly because they feel, often wrongly, there is very little room for choice or discretion in jobs in the health services. Also it may not occur to them that incorporating certain choices and flexibilities can create a much more interested, motivated and innovative work force. Stewart was not stumbling on any great or new revelation but the simple model she developed can be of great help in reviewing and re-designing jobs and work to make them much more vibrant. It is especially worthwhile to determine the real substance of the constraints in professional jobs and then to extend the space for discretion and choice as the judgements a professional ought to be able to make and the skills and knowledge they have gathered in training and experience make the room for choices very much greater than is often appreciated.

The main responsibilities for such redesign rests with the immediate manager and elements of job design are outlined in the next chapter.

The general considerations a manager should give to policies and constraints are to consider their substance and applicability to the job that is required to be done and to describe both clearly, and then to have a confidence in extending the choices he and his subordinate staff have. As the staff perform the core elements increasingly well and the more professional they are, the more room for choice exists. The manager can then use such choices and discretions to aid motivation and innovation. It is the motivating of staff and encouraging innovation that are the more practical and rewarding elements of a manager's role.

REFERENCES

1. DHSS (1977) *The Way Forward*, HMSO, London; Royal Commission on NHS (1979) *A Service for Patients*, HMSO, London; DHSS (1981) *Care in Action*, HMSO, London.
2. *NHS Management Enquiry*. Letter to Secretary of State for Social Services from R. Griffiths (leader of enquiry) 1983. (Griffiths Report).

3. McCarthy, Lord (1976) *Making Whitley Work*, DHSS, London.
4. Selwyn, N. M. (1985) *Law of Employment*, 5th edn, Butterworth, Guildford. One of the more comprehensive books on employment law.
5. Stewart, R. (1976) *Constrasts in Management*, New York, McGraw-Hill.
6. Walton, M. (1984) *Management and Managing – a Dynamic Approach*, Harper & Row, London.

Part Two

The Elements of Managing
Health Professionals

Chapter 3

Labour provisioning

Most managers have tended to be reactive in matters of personnel management. They tend to wait for a problem to arise and only then think about solving it. This is especially so in the field of the activity generally known as human resourcing or labour provisioning – obtaining, training and keeping enough skilled staff to do the job required. Many businesses and service organizations, both private and public, are very efficient at planning the type of service they aim to provide in the next two or three years – some are even very efficient at strategic planning for ten to twenty years ahead. Not so many, however, plan how, in human resource terms, they will reach their goal. Many will argue that it is too difficult to plan staffing needs with any long term precision because day-to-day and week-to-week circumstances change not only within the organization but in the labour market as a whole.

HUMAN RESOURCE PLANNING

It is well understood that time and energy spent on planning staff requirements in sufficient detail and time taken to maintain a viable stock of labour or to meet a new level of service is a worthwhile activity which can save considerable time and energy later. It is not true to say that it is so difficult to plan future staffing needs of a department or a hospital as a whole. There are a number of preconditions that need to be met but human resource or manpower planning does not need to be treated as a complex mathematical exercise.

The starting point or data base

As with most management problems the first necessity is to draw together the data and information that are relevant to the issues. In deciding what is relevant it is important to have a clear idea of the planning process [1].

The manager must first have a clear understanding of the current situation [2]. Self-evident perhaps but frequently forgotten and only if the current situation is correctly perceived is it possible to review it to determine whether any change is sensible and also what the starting point should be. The most useful data with which to set the baseline are:

Numbers of staff employed.
Permutation of full and part time.
Skill mixes including a profile of the training and experience that each member of staff has had and the permutation of qualified staff and unqualified helpers and support staff.
The costs of each type of staff.
The age structure of the staff in the department.
The turnover of staff and vacancy levels.
The current levels of sickness.
Some measure of the work done by the department and an indication of how that compares with what is reckoned to be good practice.

Such information is becoming easier to obtain now that most managers are competent in the use of micro computers which enable them to analyse a large number of different permutations. Even if a manager only analyses data for the next twelve months he will begin to get a very good idea of how many staff will retire during the period, how many are likely to leave through normal turnover and where the gaps in skills or experience are. It has been surprising that many managers until recently did not know with any degree of accuracy some basic and very useful facts such as which staff are going to retire over the next five years, what the turnover or stability rates are for their department, the level of sickness and the labour costs of each employee and for the department as a whole.

Higher productivity or more staff?

The essential element of planning at this stage is to decide whether the present stock of labour can be better used. Comparisons with other, similar, paramedical departments can be made to see where a particular department stands in a league table of productivity. The commonest measure is to compare the unit labour cost of each patient treatment [3]. This may not be very sophisticated and may not take much account of subtle (and sometimes not so subtle) elements that exist in a department such as dilapidation of buildings or equipment and case-mixes that need disproportionate time spent on them. However, it gives a baseline where in the past there may not have been one. In the health services as a whole such performance indicators [4] are becoming commonplace and although they are regarded by some as intrusive blunt instruments they do show up areas worthy of further examination. Some of the professions allied to medicine are conducting significant research into workload and patient dependency measures. In themselves they are merely interesting; taken in conjunction with planning short-term staffing, for example duty rotas, and long-term staff/skill requirements they have a great deal to offer provided they become a management tool, understood and used by managers, and not, as tends to happen, the province of those doing the research and regarded with some apprehension and mistrust by line managers.

Having decided that the present labour force is used as effectively as possible, it is necessary to analyse probable wastage. It is easy to measure wastage or turnover by the simple formula:

$$\frac{\text{Number of staff leaving in the period (normally 1 year)}}{\text{Number of staff employed at end of period}} \times 100$$

to give a percentage turnover figure. Thus, four staff who leave in a year out of a staff of twenty gives a turnover figure of 20%. Such a figure may be of help in the macro labour market but the departmental manager will need to know the nature of the turnover. Is it merely retirements or is it four people coming and going through the same job because they find the job dull or were not inducted adequately? Is it unqualified staff who are leaving or trained technical staff who may be difficult to recruit and expensive to train? Such analyses will give hints to the manager as to the nature of the problem with which he has to deal. It may in fact not be a recruitment problem he has but one of retention of staff because perhaps of poor training, low morale or bad management, which in turn are addressed in later chapters.

Planning for change

Next, the manager needs to predict future needs. This involves being clear as to the plans for the development of the service managed and translating this into requirements for different staff. It should not be merely a straight extrapolation of the present staff profile. Rather, it should be a considered analysis of how most economically and effectively the department can be developed to do additional or different work. Staffing norms have frequently been used by both health authorities and individual professions. These in effect represent average staffing levels for particular workloads. Whilst norms, like performance indicators, have their uses inasmuch as they can provide a starting point for further analysis and debate they have disadvantages. Chief amongst these are that they are historical and so might reflect moderate or even poor practice. By the same token they may not reflect trends in changing technology or clinical practice and so their use, other than a rough and ready indicator, may lead to a compounding of poor practice.

The availability of staff with particular skills has to be taken into account as do changes in technology, support services available, new techniques and any desire the manager may have to redesign the structure to give more opportunity for staff to use their own initiative. The end product of this stage, however, is a clear statement of what staff need to be recruited, promoted and trained in specified numbers over a defined period. The statement may highlight particular problems in achieving its stated goals in which case it should demonstrate ways in which those problems will be overcome. To have an unrealistic plan or one that is predictably unattainable is counterproductive as it gives the illusion of planning, control and confidence when the reverse is the case.

Supplies of labour

The third part of the process of manpower planning is to determine whether or not the labour market locally or on a wider scale can sustain the plan. The first two stages define the demand. This third stage starts to show whether the supply can meet the demand. Each of the professions, from time to time, researches and reports on the future needs for qualified staff [5] and whether the labour market can sustain such a need. In the past many of these national reports have placed a heavy emphasis on professionalization and education. They have, for example, put forward the argument that a particular profession must, for the benefit of the service and the profession itself, heighten its educational standards – often to degree standard – and consequently increase the entry qualifications. In doing so they have analysed the availability of school leavers with one or two 'A' level GCEs and decided their plans for each professional aggrandizing are practical – in short the changing demand can be met by supply. The local manager in planning the supply potential needs to go through a similar but much more local process. In this instance there is a need to examine the output of schools and colleges training basically qualified professionals, to determine whether enough of them, and more experienced professionals can be attracted to the locality or department and if there are potential difficulties in doing so to determine how such difficulties can be overcome. It might be that skill mixes can be adjusted if schools are not producing enough potential professionals; or that it would be possible to increase the attractiveness of a particular department by its reputation for post-registration training or training attachments, or by facilities for staff such as accommodation or emphasizing certain aspects of the job or locality when advertising vacant posts.

Getting planning into context

Most managers will not face the need for large-scale manpower planning more than once or twice in their careers and when they do they can normally obtain technical help from specialists. They do, however, face the continual process of labour turnover, changing clinical practices, technology and changing workload.

To cope with these they should have a plan in outline for one to two years which shows roughly how many staff and of what sort and quality they are likely to need. In addition, they should have an explicit plan of the most probable needs over the next six to nine months and a very detailed plan and programme of action for the immediate three months. The average time it takes from deciding to advertise a post to an appointee starting, let alone becoming totally effective is ten weeks even when they only need to give their current employer one month's notice. Such a programme of action will determine the level of recruitment and induction training that staff need to plan for so that those processes are performed as a routine task and not in an *ad hoc* last minute way which can be diverting to the main job in hand and often ineffectual.

Having emphasized the importance of planning it is equally important to understand that the process is not difficult as long as there is adequate information which is used in a discerning way. Further it is important not to try to get absolute precision in such planning. To do so would take far too much time and information and if circumstances changed even slightly the plan would be thrown out of gear. It is much more practical to get a plan 75% or 80% right and then start to implement it, making adjustments as one goes. The energy needed to get the last 25% or 20% element of a plan is usually significantly out of proportion to the benefit gained.

The key elements are that the manager should know the profile of the current labour force from his personnel records, should attempt to outline the general need for staff for a year or two and have detailed plans for 3–6 months ahead – normally from knowing rates of labour turnover and what service developments are likely and by way of contingency planning the manager should have a plan for covering any key job should the current job holder leave unexpectedly.

RECRUITMENT AND SELECTION

The costs of recruitment and selection decisions

If human resource planning is generally concerned with planning what staff are needed, then the recruitment, selection and induction processes are concerned with finding them and settling them into their jobs. Often, though not invariably, these processes are to do with recruiting a single employee which though not difficult takes time to do well. Experience shows that in the public sector especially, very careful and constraining procedures are set up to regulate the purchase of equipment often of no great investment value, say £500–1000. Specifications have to be written, cases of need made, tenders compiled, requisitions made out often with two or more service managers' signatures on them, detailed administrative procedures followed to the letter and the whole process is closely scrutinized by supplies or procurement departments. The average recruitment costs alone of a new member of staff are £500 (advertising, travel expenses, administrative and management time) but much more significant is the investment made in the new employee. If the average annual cost of an employee is £10 000 and they, again on average, stay in a post for five years, the investment in purely cash terms is £50 000, leaving aside the opportunity costs if the person appointed performs less than averagely. Of concern to managers must be the fact that employees who perform below the average level but are just adequate tend to stay very much longer in post so the investment and the opportunity costs are that much higher.

Specifying the job

In the past, few systems to help make such an investment wisely existed and often a *laissez-faire* attitude has been adopted as to who may decide whether a vacancy should be filled at all, if so how and who is authorized to appoint to it. Consequently little training has been given to those involved in the process although this is now beginning to change. Such changes have been very much needed in the health professions because latterly there have been two assumptions running through recruitment and selection processes. The first was that merely because someone was professionally qualified there was a presumption of skill and appropriateness for a particular post; such a presumption is not automatically justified. The second assumption has been more difficult to change; it was that a manager of professional staff, merely because he had been appointed as a manager, had a high level of skill in the recruitment and selection process. Without such skill and knowledge it is probable that the manager will depend on inherent views, attitudes and prejudices, all of which lead to subjective decisions. With knowledge and skill, together with some system or drill to work to, greater levels of objectivity can be brought to bear, although no infallible system of recruitment and selection has yet been devised.

The process is about getting properly shaped pegs into holes of a prescribed shape. Such a process must begin by being very clear on the shape of the hole. In outline the most logical order of going about things is:

- to decide that a job needs to be filled. This decision will have been arrived at through the manpower planning work that will have previously been done, unless an unexpected vacancy crops up. It must be clear who makes that decision; it may well be a more senior manager who is not necessarily involved in the rest of the process.
- to design the job. This also may have been a part of the earlier planning activity – the end product will normally be a job description.
- to devise largely from the job description a person specification.
- to attract a field of appropriate applicants.
- to screen and shortlist the applicants.
- to test and interview the candidates shortlisted.
- to make an offer and confirm the appointment.
- to induct the appointee.

This is a traditional order but it has so far stood the test of time and is on balance the most economic, effective and fair way of recruiting.

Designing and defining the job

Whilst the fundamental component of any job description is an outline of the duties and responsibilities required of the job holder it should be used to satisfy a number of other needs.

The interaction of jobs and levels
When designed, the job needs to fit into the pattern of other jobs in the department. Strict lines of demarcation can create

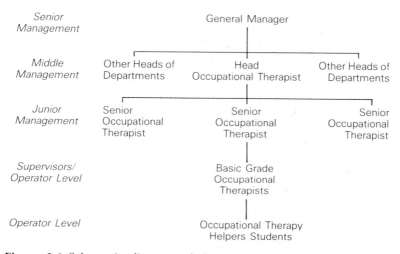

Figure 3.1 Schematic diagram of the organizational structure of a typical Occupational Therapy Department.

problems as many managers during the 1950s and 1960s could testify. Each job, however, has a uniqueness. It is there to make a defined contribution to the enterprise, if it does not it is not needed. In addition, it depends on the jobs around it, as they depend on it, and those dependencies need to be recognized in its design. So too do the different levels of responsibility that accrue to different jobs so that they can be placed in the most appropriate level in the hierarchy and so that fair grades or levels of pay can be awarded to the posts. This position of a post in an organization can be described schematically. This has the advantage of showing the size of the organization as well as which posts are responsible to which supervisors and managers. Typically an organization chart for, say, an Occupational Therapy department would be as in Fig. 3.1.

Such a schematic chart though not always essential can be of great help in assisting the analysis and definition of component parts of the job description. Prescribing the degree of autonomy and authority can be aided by such a chart especially if the overall manager is trying to increase the degree of choice for job holders at each level. If he decides on a change at one level the chart can be used as a checklist to help determine the effects of that change throughout the structure. Such changes may be to do with technical or professional work or be a redefinition of managerial or supervisory responsibilities. Either way such statements of definition must be clear and unambiguous.

Individual job design

When describing the duties and responsibilities, there is a temptation to go into too much detail of not only what must be done but how it should be done. For professionally based jobs such a catalogue of detail is not only unnecessary but can be counter-productive especially if innovation is to be encouraged. An outline of what the job is in existence to do – its overall purpose – needs two or three lines at the most and then five or six key areas of responsibility need to be listed together with an outline of the general standard of performance that is expected. A key area of responsibility or task would be one which contributes substantially to the success of the post and is defined in a measurable way. It should be about what needs to be done and not how the job holder is expected to do his job. In any event it is much more practical to set measurable standards of performance on the objects which a job is set up to achieve rather than how they are achieved.

A job description is beginning to be out of date as soon as it is written. It follows that minute detail will tend to get in the way of progress in any organization where techniques of work or the organization of work change and difficulties are compounded when such changes are rapid. The job description is not part of the contract of employment unless it goes into such detail that it is seen to be implicitly so or unless there is an express term to state so. The job description should go into just enough detail to identify the employee's main responsibilities but be general enough to allow variations to take place in duties and tasks within the contract of employment. It is useful to remember that tasks and duties, like contracts, are negotiable and can be changed by agreement.

A major part of the management process is the continuous review of work, resetting objectives and adjusting duties, responsibilities and tasks. A job description should allow for such changes to take place.

It is usually of great help to outline the key tasks needed in the job. This tells applicants what is expected as well as assisting the manager in drawing up a person specification as an aid to selection. Similarly the conditions in which the job is to be done may warrant description especially if, for example, there are any environmental elements or conditions that are unusual or might not otherwise be expected such as an obligation to live within 15 minutes' travelling time of the hospital to meet on-call commitments.

Clauses such as . . .' and any other duties that may be decided' and . . .' this job description may be reviewed at a later date' are both unnecessary in that both will or ought to happen and can be expected by the applicant in the normal course of events. The first phrase in particular merely serves to demonstrate that the author of the job description may not have given proper thought to it. A typical format for a job description would be:

1. Job title (this should say what it means);
2. Responsible to;
3. Purpose of job or outline of role;
4. Key responsibilities (five or six);
5. Key skills required;
6. Major conditions of work;
7. Major conditions of service (including grade or rate of pay).

The job description for, say, a superintendent physiotherapist post might look like:

Post/Job title: Superintendent Physiotherapist – general hospital

Responsible to: District Physiotherapist

Purpose of job:
To ensure the effective and professional management development of physiotherapy services within the hospital.

Key responsibilities:
1. To ensure the effective management of the physiotherapy service, its staff and its budget.
2. To set and achieve specified standards of service in conjunction with users of the service.
3. Plans the development of the service in liaison with users of the service and other professional groups.

4. Is responsible for the review of all staff's performance and ensures their training and development is in accord with their needs as well as the aims of the department.
5. Develops systems to monitor the efficacy of staffing and financial expenditure and to determine the optimum work-load within given resources.
6. Ensures management and clinical policies are implemented. Amends and reviews these as appropriate.

Key skills required:
The post holder must be a Chartered Physiotherapist and have at least eight years' hospital physiotherapy experience of which four must be in posts involving significant management and planning experience.

Major conditions of work:
This job is based within the hospital and has no management responsibilities outside it. The department itself is modern and fully equipped. Most of the wards are modern although some, which are soon to be replaced, are dilapidated, cramped and difficult to work in.

Major conditions of service:
The post holder will have his/her own case load amounting to approximately half time. The grade for this post is Superin-tendent Physiotherapist I. The working week is Monday to Friday but all staff participate in out-of-hours and weekend duty to provide an on-call service. Other conditions are as outlined in P and T Whitley Council.

Specifying the qualities needed – the person specification

Having defined the nature of the job and some of the major conditions that are part of it, before advertising for someone to fill the post it has always been useful to specify the qualities of the person who will fit the bill. In recent years with increasing emphasis on equal opportunity and with most employers trying to eliminate forms of discrimination, the person specification takes on a much more crucial role. [6] It becomes a tool that encourages a manager to be much more analytical and objective in the qualities genuinely required of a person. In that way it becomes not only easier to design advertising material but also to test applicants against objective criteria. Subsequent to the appointment it becomes easier to justify the decision, if called upon to do so, by demonstrating that the criteria were met by the successful applicant and not, or not to the same degree, by those who were unsuccessful. In devising the job description most of the work for deriving a person specification has been done. It need only be brief and in a format that helps the actual shortlisting, testing and/or interviewing of the applicants. The most practical method to adopt is a systematic one and a number have been developed. Examples are the Five Fold Framework developed by John Munro Fraser [7] and the now much more frequently used Seven Point Plan [8]. Both systems aim to help a manager list the characteristics and qualities that have to be taken into account in an individual in the context of a particular job.

The seven headings used in the Seven Point Plan are:

1. Physical Make-up
   What degree of strength, state of health, appearance, are required in a person to do the job?
2. Attainments
   What is the minimum (and desirable) level of education, specialist or professional training, previous experience, e.g. of basic grade work or supervision/management required?
3. General Intelligence
   What level and nature of intelligence is needed to do the job well? This is to do with problem-solving ability or in jobs involving a lot of initiative and lateral thinking.
4. Special Aptitudes
   What special aptitudes or skills does the job demand, e.g. manual dexterity or particular degree of verbal or written articulateness?
5. Interests
   Does the job call for particular interests in certain areas?
6. Disposition
   Is it a requirement of the job holder to be able to get on with people, lead others, be reliable, be adaptable?
7. Circumstances
   Is it necessary for the job holder to travel; how influenced by pay or status might an applicant be?

In compiling a person specification for a particular job each subject heading needs to be considered and only the qualities really needed in a successful applicant to do the job prescribed. A lax analysis of these qualities can considerably reduce the objectivity a more thorough or thoughtful analysis would give. Such laxity can lead to discrimination which may lack moral validity, could break the law and certainly will create potential waste or inefficiency in the selection process. An example might be that a manager feels adaptability and enthusaism are, possibly quite correctly, crucial characteristics in a future post holder. Because of the manager's laxness and possibly because of his conditioning and stereotyping he assumes only young people have those qualities so under one heading or another he enters 'essential age range 25–35' and may make no mention of the real qualities required which may be present in people less than 25 or over 35. In one phrase, in that specification he has reduced his chance of recruiting someone with all the necessary qualities by a factor of four.

Using the job description already devised for the Superintendent Physiotherapist it is how possible to compile a person specification for the post:

Person Specification

Job title: Superintendent Physiotherapist I		
		Essential or desirable? (E or D)
1. Physical make-up	Physically fit other than certain disabilities, e.g. limited sight handicap, controlled epilepsy.	E
2. Attainments	Chartered Physiotherapist.	E
	Experience of all hospital physiotherapy specialties.	D
	Management experience in a large hospital department.	E
	Management training.	E
3. General intelligence	Ability to analyse the nature of medium scale issues.	E

	Ability to stand above and view all the component parts of complex issues.	D
	Evidence that such abilities have been used.	E/D
4. Special aptitudes	Professional manual/ manipulative skills.	E
	Verbally articulate.	E
	Numerate – to the point of being able to analyse departmental data.	E
5. Interests	Interest in the development of the profession.	D
	Rehabilitation generally.	D
6. Disposition	Acceptable to peer groups and colleagues.	E
	Influencing skills.	D
	Leadership ability in respect of small groups.	E
	Dependable and thorough.	D
	Flexible/adaptable.	D
7. Circumstances	Stable.	D
	Realistically ambitious.	D

Attracting a field of applicants

There are a number of ways of attracting the type of applicants a manager is seeking such as head hunting, keeping a waiting list, asking existing staff if they know of anyone suitable, promoting from within or rotating staff through posts. However, the most usual and probably the most efficient and fair way of attracting applicants to posts is to advertise. Additionally, most public health services have recruitment policies which make advertising most posts mandatory. This should certainly be the case, given the present health service culture and desire for open management, where the vacant post might involve promotion for applicants. Generally speaking, advertisements appear in newspapers or professional journals. There are many other forms, including radio, television, local bulletins, advertising in local post offices and the sides of buses. Writing copy for advertising is a skill that can be learned quite easily but often can be left, for administrative ease to a specialist.

A number of elements, however, are important. Basic information about the post should be outlined including job title, level or pay, key qualities required in applicants (this also has the virtue of helping to filter out inappropriate potential applicants by self-selection), a very brief description of the job and work place if these are not apparent in the job title and address for responses, a contact point for more information, clear instructions on how and where to apply and a closing date.

The need for an elaborate and potentially costly advertisement will depend on the manager's judgement of the labour market, the number of posts that are being advertised and the impression or image desired. An advertisement may have a non-recruitment spin-off in that it projects the image of the organization to a wider audience than just those who may be looking for a job. At a time when health service employers are becoming much more aware of their obligation to consumers and the public at large, job advertisements give a further medium for presenting a higher general profile. In general, however, it is usually more effective to target advertising as closely as possible. For this reason for particular professional posts it is usually best, and cheapest, to use the professional press. Moreover there may well be local national policies on the format and medium for advertisements and these will need to be understood and complied with.

The ideal response to an advertisement is a few applicants of high quality and not a vast number, all of which need consideration and considerable administrative work. Respondents to advertisements need to be dealt with courteously, positively and in good time – the employing manager often needs them more than they need him. In fact advertising should not only be aimed at those who actively want a change of job, it should equally try to tempt those who feel quite happy where they currently are and have not yet thought of a move.

An essential part of the good treatment of respondents is the information they are given. Clearly the job description should be sent but so, too, should further advice or information on the job, the department and its plans for the future, the facilities for further training, and an outline of the locality. Applicants need to be advised on what will happen if they apply. Do they fill in a standard application form or should they send a curriculum vitae; do they know when interviews will take place and will they be told if they are shortlisted in good time?

Screening and shortlisting

When screening and shortlisting a field of applicants no applicant should be shortlisted unless their application form gives a good indication that they have all the qualities, as determined by the person specification, to do the job. It is invariably misconceived and often discourteous and hurtful to shortlist an inappropriate applicant to make up the numbers for interview or because he/she is an internal applicant. It is also wasteful of the organization's time. There can be no rigid guidance as to the numbers shortlisted but for one job no more than three or four should be called for interview if each is to be given enough time for recruiter and applicant to find out enough about each other.

It is at this point that a well-constructed person specification comes into its own, especially if the application form is well designed using a similar format. It is a relatively simple matter, with practice, to set one form alongside the other and compare the two. The only other skill needed is to interpret certain entries on an application form that will clearly have been written to show the applicant in the best possible light; and to spot significant or unexplained gaps in employment, experience or education and training. It is advisable, for review and monitoring purposes, to make brief notes of why applicants have or have not been shortlisted. The same applies at the interview stage. Such monitoring should be put to good use inside the organization to improve selection systems and may be of help to show outside agencies, such as the Equal Opportunities Commission, success in eliminating discrimination [6].

Testing and interviewing

Of these two techniques, which are not mutually exclusive, interviewing is the one that is used the most. In fact in the health services there is a marked reluctance to put a job applicant through almost any form of test. The reasons for such reluctance are not altogether clear but are probably because testing is still regarded as not quite the proper thing to do amongst professionals and the skills and knowledge needed for some tests take time to acquire. Some forms of testing, for example personality and psychometric testing, need very specialist skills to conduct otherwise not only will the results be unhelpful but positive damage may be done. The main qualities that can be tested for are intelligence or general mental capacity, particular aptitudes such as adaptability or resilience, professional or manual skills and certain elements of personality [9].

This section does not set out to describe all the forms of test that can be applied [10]. It does aim, however, to give managers a confidence or at least an initial enthusiasm to use tests where they are appropriate. From the job description and person specification for a shorthand typist it should be clear that the job holder must be able to take shorthand and to type. Both these qualities are easily tested but it is a matter of constant surprise and some concern how rarely a recruiter does in fact test for them and merely accepts at face value that an applicant can take shorthand at 100 words per minute and type at 60.

Similarly, it is possible to test for many attributes in the professional and technical fields. Manual skills can be tested physically and mental or thinking qualities can be tested by case studies asking applicants to make presentations or to write a report as well as at the traditional interview. The important point to bear in mind is that if a particular quality is important in a job and is testable, then test it. It is, however, proper to let candidates know that there will be a test of one sort or another otherwise they may be thrown off balance which would reduce the validity of the test. Also as testing is relatively rare it would be discourteous to confront a candidate with a test on the day of interview without prior notice.

Interviewing and some of the pitfalls

The interview is still the most common process used for selection and is likely to remain so. Certainly no appointment should be made without an interview for otherwise it becomes difficult for both candidate and manager to form any judgement on a large number of skills and attributes. The interview is also an ideal process in which to test the veracity and applicability of what is on the application form and whether candidate and manager will get on with each other to the extent that is needed in the job. Most managers, and indeed candidates, see the interview as the focus of the selection process. Most interviewers, however, are not as expert as they believe and very few set aside adequate time to prepare for the interview.

One of the main attributes of a good interview is that the interviewer gets on the same wavelength as the candidate. He is unlikely to do this if he has not read the application form, thoroughly understood the job description, given thought to the line of questioning and planned in outline the format of the interview so that all the major subject areas are covered by both interviewer and candidate. The interviewer also needs to plan how much not to say. There is a strong tendency amongst interviewers to talk too much rather than to draw the candidate out. At interviews of professional candidates personal experience shows that as much as 75% of the time has been taken up by the interviewers talking, leaving only a quarter of the time for the candidate to put his case. Ten minutes worth of candidate's responses is hardly a good basis for making a selection investment decision.

The interviewer must be aware of his own prejudices. The unbiased interviewer does not exist but a good one recognizes his biases and for all practical purposes excludes them. Not to do so creates obvious results, some of which might bring about claims of illegal discrimination and most of which will result in a decision being made that is less effective than might have been. The halo effect [6], first identified before World War II, needs to be borne in mind and is manifest when a favourable generalization about a candidate's overall ability or personality is judged by the interviewer on the basis of only one quality possessed by the candidate. Often such a quality is one towards which the interviewer has a special leaning. An example might be that a low sickness record is taken as an indicator that the candidate is a hard worker who produces good work.

The biggest danger to be aware of, however, is that most of us are more predisposed to someone who is likeable and there is a major tendency to ascribe many qualities to someone we like. People we like we tend to see as more intelligent, harder working, more adaptable, and more discerning. In short we impute good or worthy qualities to someone we find likeable or attractive. If the person specification suggests such qualities are important in the job they should be tested or validated positively during the interview – not merely assumed. Again personal experience shows that the selection and appointment of large numbers of supervisory and management staff in the health professions have been very largely on the basis that applicants got on with people or more often that they were good at their former, basic job. On this basis it was assumed they would be effective managers. Such assumptions carry great risk if the applicant's managerial potential is not tested specifically at interview or by some test or presentation.

The prime function of the interview is to determine whether by past achievement the interviewer can predict future performance of the interviewee and in so doing decide who is the best candidate for the job. This being so there are a number of useful tenets to observe:

First, plan a format for the interview so that all important facts are covered. If there is more than one interviewer, make sure each knows the area they are to cover and give each long enough to create some empathy with the candidate. The interview is not an inquisition – there is little to be said for using stress interview techniques in recruiting professional staff – so while an interviewer should be firm and get answers to questions as asked, there is no call for aggression or blustering.

Second, the interview should be seen as very much a two-way process with the candidate being drawn out to do his share of the responding and if necessary the questioning. At the end a negotiated bargain – a contract – is going to be struck and each party needs to be as sure as possible that they know what they are bargaining for.

Third, if the candidate is to be drawn out, open questions should be asked. These call for a measured, well-argued response or comment and not merely a 'yes' or 'no' answer.

Fourth, the questions should elicit clarity on points of doubt in the application form. It is useful to have as the basis of questions the main qualities called for in the person specification. This gives a form and sense of purpose to the interview and a basis for making a judgement when the interview is concluded.

Fifth, avoid questions that involve direct or indirect discrimination. Questions such as 'are you thinking of starting a family' or 'have you made provision for your children' are often asked of women. Even if they are asked of male candidates as well they may still be discriminatory because the conditioned reaction to the answer is influenced by the gender of the respondent. In any event answers to such questions fail to give a full or accurate picture; one can imagine a candidate being asked if she has made proper provision for her children (a closed question anyway) and answering 'yes' only to find subsequently that she has a horse which has to be fed and she cannot get to work before 9 a.m. She could with some rectitude turn round and say she was never asked about her horse! If an interviewer is trying to find out how committed the candidate is to the job or whether his attendance pattern is going to be adequate, there are ways of finding out by examining past performance, references, or by asking whether the candidate fully understands the work pattern of the department.

Sixth, the interviewers need to listen to what the applicant is saying and not, as is often the temptation, start thinking of the next question.

If the interview is going to produce effective results, the number of interviewers must be kept down. There is rarely a case to be made for more than three interviewers and the ideal for creating a balance between thoroughness and empathy with the candidate is two. If a manager wants to involve more people than three the most practical way is to have some individual interviews before the final panel interview in which such extra interviewers can participate.

The number of candidates interviewed should not be more than three or four. When there are more than four either not enough time is given to each or interviewers get tired or jaded or sometimes even forget, if they have not made notes, which candidate said what and left what impression. Such qualities are not conducive to a good decision.

An interview is a formal process and it should never be assumed it is not. It is for the panel to decide how to conduct the interview but they should have in mind the need to put the candidate at ease. This may entail an informal atmosphere or layout of furniture and an apparently relaxed method of questioning but the candidate will certainly see the process as formal so the interviewers should recognize this. At the end of the interview the candidates must have had the chance to say what they wanted to or to clarify any points of uncertainty. They must also be clear what is going to happen. They need to know when a decision will be made and how it will be made known, just as the interviewer may want to know if a candidate is still interested in the job.

Because of the importance of the interview and the, often, limited experience and skill many managers have in the process, it is essential that before any interviewing is done the proposed interviewer is trained. This helps give the appropriate knowledge and some basic skills which can then be practised. Also, and more importantly in the early days it gives the interviewer a confidence that is crucial if the interviews are to be conducted effectively.

Whatever the outcome, especially with professional groups, the unsuccessful candidates particularly should go away with the feeling that they have been treated fairly and sensitively and with the thought that they would very much like to work for the organization even though on this occasion it has rejected them.

APPOINTMENT AND MAKING A START

The job offer

An offer of a job should only be made if there is confidence that the applicant can do the job and is the best candidate available. It may be felt expedient to appoint a second-rate applicant merely to fill a gap but such a decision will usually be regretted later.

The main terms and conditions of the offer should be clear and if the candidate accepts the offer a contract exists. It is, however, wise to confirm the appointment in writing explicitly detailing the conditions the contract is subject to, for example, a satisfactory medical examination. If such a condition applies, it is only fair not to expect the appointee to ratify his acceptance or hand in his notice to his current employer until the outcome is known. It can never be acceptable to make an appointment subject to references as to do so can cause a breach of confidence when, for example, the offer is withdrawn after poor references are available. References should be available at or before interview and any lack of clarity resolved with the referee before any offer of appointment is made.

The final points are to agree a starting date and make sure the new member of staff is clear about joining instructions.

Induction and settling in

Left to their own devices, more new staff leave an organization or get into bad habits in the first six months than in any other period of their employment. Both factors cause organization problems and cost a great deal and both are avoidable.

Induction training is an element of personnel management that almost all agree is a good thing but not many do well. The aim of induction is to ease the new employee comfortably into the organization by making them aware immediately of knowledge needed from the outset and helping them progressively to know the factors that will be needed in their medium- and long-term work.

Immediate matters to be dealt with are usually of a practical nature and easily overlooked. Knowing how to obtain a uniform; understanding fire and safety rules; knowing how to get meals; understanding the most important policies and procedures of the department, especially personnel policies and rules; knowing about on-call arrangements and working rotas. Slightly longer term needs will include matters such as understanding the organizational structure and the policies and procedures of less immediate application. Often it can be helpful to agree an induction programme with the new employee so that real needs are satisfied. This avoids the situation where an impersonal check list is unthinkingly followed. Too many induction programmes involve the new employee in spending his first full week or fortnight meeting a steady stream of managers and other personalities in the organization with whom he may, or may not, have some future contact. This is usually a mistake. Most people only need to know those people and facts that are of immediate impact and then want to get on with the job. Meeting the more distant people can come in the second or third phase by which time the new member of staff can exercise his own discretion to a much greater degree.

The employee's manager is the key person and the one who is responsible for this easing-in period. He should spend time outlining the immediate structure, procedures and tasks for the employee and checking that the employee understands what he has been told. Although checklists have a value – mainly as an *aide-mémoire* – they can be used too mechanistically by the manager who sees the functions listed as a chore to be checked off on a list in order to demonstrate that he has done his job. It follows that most induction training will be organized by the manager. There is a case for some induction training to be mounted more centrally to tap particular expertise and to gain economies of scale. Such training would be in the secondary phase and be organized as frequently as the number of new staff in a hospital or group of departments required it. The content would need to be of interest and relevance to all those attending and might consist of a talk or discussion on the size and complexity of the hospital, what its main activities are, what the plans for it are, an outline of the overall organization and who is who, an insight into broadbrush policies such as those which apply to public relations, the image of the hospital and the way it sees itself serving the community.

Most organized induction programmes fall into disrepair because they are run routinely in a mechanistic way with more emphasis given to running them than to the needs of the new staff who do not see them as being particularly useful and so a vicious circle starts. The essence and benefit of good induction come from the needs of the new employee being clearly recognized and satisfied by the immediate manager. The manager should not rely passively on central courses but where these are useful he should demand that he makes a contribution or at the least that the real training needs are satisfied. Future induction training can usually be improved by asking past participants for their comments. Such a review should not be time consuming or sophisticated but if a member of staff has something to say, as with all subjects, he should be listened to.

If everything has gone according to plan a new member of staff has been efficiently recruited, selected, appointed and has settled into his job. Following the processes described cannot guarantee success. People with quirks and personalities are involved and judgements have to be made at each stage of the recruitment and selection process. Such points, however, reinforce the need for a systematic approach in order to inject some order and objectivity into what would otherwise be a very hit and miss exercise. With the stakes being so high the more order and objectivity that can be achieved the more the outcome will improve. In terms of the staff management of the employee, however, the journey has only just begun. A phase of two or three months is over. The next phase, that of developing, motivating, organizing and controlling, which will hopefully last two or three years at least and possibly a working lifetime, has just begun.

REFERENCES

1. Bramham, J. (1975) *Practical Manpower Planning*, Institute of Personnel Management, London.
2. Singer, E. J. and Ramsden, J. (1972) *Human Resources. Obtaining Results from People at Work*, McGraw-Hill, London.
3. Stainer, G. (1971) *Manpower Planning – the Management of Human Resources*, Heinemann, London.
4. DHSS Performance Indicators Group (1987) *Performance Indicators for the NHS Manpower*, DHSS, London.
5. CPSM (1979) *The Next Decade*, CPSM, London, United Kingdom Central Council for Nursing, Midwifery and Health Visiting (1987) *Project 2000 – Counting the Cost*, UKCC, London.
6. Commission for Racial Equality (1984) *Code of Practice*, London; Equal Opportunities Commission (1985) *Guide for Employers*, EOC, London.
7. Fraser, J. M. (1971) *Introduction to Personnel Management*, Nelson, London.
8. Rodger, A. (1952) *The Seven Point Plan*, National Institute of Industrial Psychology, London.
9. Edwardes, M. (1983) *Back from the Brink*, Collins, London.
10. *Psychological Assessment* (1985) IDS Study 341. Income Data Service Ltd, London.

Chapter 4

Motivation and leadership

The bulk of a manager's job is involved in getting other people to do the work that is needed by the organization in the most economic and effective way. Despite this fact many managers have never studied the subject of what makes people tick, what makes them enthusiastic, efficient and hard working and so it is hardly surprising that many employees are not encouraged to give of their best. This state of affairs continues to exist despite the fact that the health business has some of the best intrinsic motivating factors that could be hoped for in any business. These factors are mainly at the more noble end of the human behaviour spectrum – altruism, a sense of belonging to a skilled profession, a sense of vocation and looking after those less fortunate than oneself and being held in high esteem by patients in particular and the public generally.

MOTIVATIONAL FORCES

Perhaps it is because such factors are so apparent that many managers of health professionals have not bothered too much with motivating and leading their workforce, or have ignored some of the more basic and prosaic motivational factors. History shows that many of the professions allied to medicine have pay rates that are relatively low, partly because they are often largely composed of women but also because pay claims, over a long period, have been mollified by a sense of vocation felt by the staff groups involved. Ignoring the fundamental motivational factors or trading them off against more ethereal factors is a recipe for long-term decay of any profession – a fact that a number are now beginning to recognize.

Elements of motivation

Since 1955 a significant number of theories on motivation at work have been formulated. Many of them add elements to our understanding of how employees respond to different stimuli and influences at work. Many of these theories tend to put forward specific hypotheses which tends to limit them to examining fairly specific decision making situations such as where an individual is making a choice between two activities [1].

A more general theory for understanding motivation at work was propounded by Maslow [2], more than thirty years ago. He formulated a model which put a human being's needs in general, though more particularly at work, into a hierarchy. His message was simple in that the basic needs of individuals must be satisfied before higher level factors can be considered. If this is not done, significant tensions can be generated, creating disruption or at best limiting productivity. The hierarchy is composed of five main levels which can be illustrated simply as a triangle (Fig. 4.1):

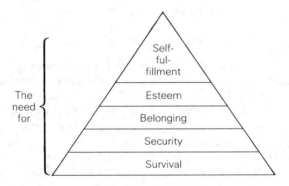

Figure 4.1 Maslow's hierarchy of needs.

First to be satisfied is the basic need for survival such as food and shelter.

Second is the need for safety, knowing that survival is not threatened, at work this is manifest in a desire for security.

Third are the social needs, a sense of belonging and being accepted by one's colleagues.

Fourth is the need to be held in high esteem and having a belief in one's significance.

Finally there is the need for self-fulfilment which entails expanding one's own horizons and by fulfilling all one's personal aims.

There are some people for whom it takes little to satisfy some of the lower order factors and for whom the higher order ones are much more important. Poets and artists will starve in garrets to get artistic kudos or self-fulfilment but most people in more mundane forms of life and employment need a great deal more satisfying in the lower factors. A manager needs to be sensitive to the degree to which a particular factor is, or needs to be, satisfied before having to consider the next level. Such progression is important because it is a human trait that they are motivationally dynamic, in that once satisfied in one sphere (as long as that satisfaction continues) people need a new stimulus.

MOTIVATING HEALTH PROFESSIONALS

Coping with unilateralism

The local manager can learn quite a lot from Maslow's model in recognizing that in most employment spheres at least the first two levels of need are almost automatically satisfied. It follows that more attention can then be given to welding a team together, creating a sense of belonging or cohesion. The need for a manager to give attention to these levels becomes especially marked in groups that have a sense of vocation and professionalism. In such groups there is a tendency to believe that the work they do and the way in which they do it is crucial and more important than most other groups. Such a unilateralist view will cause rifts if it is not ameliorated and made part of the overall business. Whilst this must be done in a way that does not destroy the energy that comes from professional independence and elitism, it needs to be done to ensure a smooth working total structure. The best way in which this can be done is to ensure that groups and individuals are committed first and foremost to the overall goals of the business and see their role as a contribution to that rather than an end in itself. Evidence available in the health services shows that when this is not achieved, major conflicts between professions can erupt, as was the case from 1974 (to the present day in some areas) between medical laboratory scientific officers and medically qualified pathologists.

Citing theories or models, however, may give the impression that if they are followed or used then staff motivation will be achieved. Such a view is simplistic. People, whether at work or not, and more especially when they are in groups, are highly complex. They have moods and they can act, depending on one's viewpoint, abnormally or irrationally. Such behaviour patterns are more likely to exist in large, complex and impersonal organizations, such as district general hospitals, unless the managers concerned are aware of and reasonably skilled in motivation and leadership.

Motivational styles

The way in which a manager will motivate staff will depend on more than just a knowledge of motivational factors; the method of managing and how the manager is perceived are important. The management style of the nineteenth and early twentieth centuries tended to be autocratic or dictatorial. Such styles were based on the notion that the manager was the owners' representative, had 'come up the hard way', knew best and had an inherent right to be obeyed. The caricature of the autocratic mill owner must have been quite near the truth and in the circumstances of the time and culture, worked to a point. Such a style is now regarded by most as restricting and limiting to initiative, ideas and energy. If there was an advantage in such a style it was that lines of communication and responsibility were clear, although such qualities are capable of being created within most management styles. Autocracy also can easily create resentment and consequent conflict. In certain circumstances orders have to be obeyed without question and such a style can exist in a hospital, for instance in an operating theatre. The professional health worker here will know what his job is, knows why he is there and knows he must be co-ordinated or instructed by the surgeon. Whilst such a scenario could spawn an autocratic style, and has done so, it is not inevitable and frequently a style more akin to team working is engendered.

If an autocratic style is based on rigid control then the other end of the spectrum is the laid back or *laissez-faire* way of doing things – or often not getting them done. Such a style is exemplified by allowing things to happen, hoping that all will turn out all right in the end. The result is that staff do not know what is expected of them, there is no clear idea of what the department or organization is in business for or what its aims and priorities might be. It may seem an attractive proposition to some but the lack of a *raison d'être* and the resulting uncertainty will soon bring about confusion, lethargy and low morale.

The present culture in society and the labour market points to some intermediate style as being the most propitious. Where on the spectrum a manager or employing organization sets its style will depend on the organization's own culture. The degree of independent professionalism that exists in the organization, whether it is a process manufacturing or a service organization will influence this decision. Similarly, whether the organization is relatively static technologically or is in the forefront of research and development activity will have a bearing on the management style which is adopted.

The fundamental element of motivating and leading work groups, especially those in the health professions where a degree of skill and professional autonomy is present, is involvement or having a style that is participative. This being so the manager needs to lean towards a democratic way of working, as long as this is in general and genuine sympathy with his own personality. He will then genuinely involve his staff in the business of the department. Tensions will begin to arise if a style is adopted that is out of balance with the predilections, culture and abilities of the manager and the staff. There needs to be recognition that staff as a whole and as individuals have a great deal of skill, knowledge and experience which could and should be put to good use. The manager who adopts a democratic, participative style tries to generate a climate in which each member of staff can express views, put forward ideas, criticize and comment or even dissent without being worried about being seen as disloyal by the manager or ridiculed or rejected by his colleagues. If such participation is genuine, and seen as such, morale tends to rise and individuals become more involved in and committed to their own job and the role of the wider work group. A manager in such a group will tend to be regarded as the *primus inter pares* whose main tasks are co-ordination, encouraging participation, initiating training and ensuring the group reviews its progress and work.

To build up a department's morale and culture in a participative and involving style in good times is relatively easy and problem free. The significant achievement is for the participative process to be genuinely available to help a department through bad times. This will mean that a manager has to be genuine in his style otherwise when major problems arise he may revert to a type that is largely autocratic; not only does confusion follow at a time when it is most destructive, but subordinate staff see him for what he really is. A genuinely participative approach does not preclude the need for decisiveness in a manager. Such decisiveness, however, needs to accrue from competence, consistency of action and style and trust. In effect this means that staff consent, explicitly or implicitly, to being managed in a particular way which at times will mean being told or asked to do something, sometimes without there having been much discussion.

The character, personality and beliefs of the manager cannot be ignored. If he is what McGregor [3] would term a Theory X Manager he would believe that work is inherently distasteful, people are lazy, not ambitious and not creative but need rigid control, then his style would lean towards being autocratic. If, however, he is a Theory Y Manager, that is one who believes work is natural, people can be creative and imaginative at work if the climate is right, can control and organize themselves quite well, then he will tend to be a participative or democratic manager. Neither style is wrong. Different shades are more appropriate to particular departments, industries and professions and the choice of shade is to some extent the organization's as a corporate body and to some extent the individual manager's.

Lessons and prerequisites in motivation

A great deal of theoretical and empirical research has been conducted in motivation much of which in general terms is consistent with Maslow's model. One of the most interesting and frequently cited is the Hawthorne study. Experiments were initiated at the Western Electric Company at their Hawthorne works in Chicago sixty years ago [4]. The studies included investigating the effects on output of factors such as temperature, lighting, length of working day, number and length of breaks. The research was done in a specially built room and, progressively, conditions were improved and output improved. However, when some of the improved conditions were removed, output did not fall to its original levels. Studies showed that a much more involved and favourable attitude to work had evolved. Issues were discussed amongst the workers, who in turn felt freer to express views and put forward ideas. Co-operation increased and workers, more and more, began to control their own work, absence from work dropped and output continued to rise. The experiments also showed that the work group and the factory as a whole were societies in themselves as well as being a microcosm of a larger society. If attention is paid to its members, their experience used and ideas sought they become, and feel, more involved and committed to what they are doing. The main results of the experiments, which have many lessons today for managers, are that the work and productivity of staff and the social functions of management are very closely linked and most especially if managers show regard for, and encourage the involvement of, staff the attitude of those staff to the department or the organization as a whole improves. Key to the improvements was also the fact that the culture and cohesion of the work group was used and developed; to have broken the whole group up and to have worked against its culture would probably have caused a deterioration in attitude and a rift between management and staff.

A number of lessons can be learned from the experiments. Many have been confirmed by subsequent research or experience and the more important are:

- managers need to be in tune with the culture and norms of the work groups they manage.
- managers need to recognize the strong links between attitude of staff, productivity and their own management style.
- that involvement and participation, as well as improved

facilities, improve the attitudes of staff and through that comes improved output in terms of both quantity and quality.

The role of the manager in promoting such a change in attitudes is crucial for without cohesion and initiatives coming at least to start with from above, it is likely that any changes will be badly organized, uncontrolled and ill timed. It is not merely techniques of managing the people that are important but the very essence and style of leadership. Management styles have been discussed so some attention to the elements of leadership is needed.

LEADERSHIP AS A MOTIVATOR

Elements of managerial leadership

First, there has to be recognition that the manager is competent. Often this is seen as being an ability to do the jobs of all those managed as well as or even better than those who are paid to do them. A frequent statement made by managers is . . . 'I would not ask a member of staff to do a job I could not do . . .' Such a statement is impractical and points to a misundertanding of leadership. The true essence is that the manager understands what subordinate staff do, how what each of them does relates with the others, and ensures they have the wherewithal to do their work. If it were true that a manager had to be able to do all that his subordinates could do, then no management structure, especially those involving clinical and professional staff could ever work. Few would expect a doctor to be able to do the detailed work of a nurse, physiotherapist or occupational thera-pist. The doctor would be expected to know broadly what each of them did but as professionals they control the detail and more importantly how they do their work. However, promotion into management posts is still often based on the fact that the person has been good at the basic job and it must follow some-how that they will be able to manage similar workers simply for that reason. An element of this may be true but it has already been seen that managing people needs very different qualities, skills and knowledge than those that are needed to do the technicalities of a basic job. The competence that a manager must be seen to possess is the ability to manage people who have professional skills; an appreciation of their professional skills and the contribution they make is important in this but not exclusive.

Secondly, there is the quality of leading by example. By doing so the manager may demonstrate professional or managerial skill but again it is easy to align the need for such a characteristic with that of having to be able to do the job of all subordinate staff. True leadership by example is developed by the manager setting standards and then ensuring that everything is done to that level and expecting and demanding similar standards from subordinate staff in the work they do. For some managers, ability to show such a standard in a particular piece of professional work is important and is totally valid. It would be a mistake for a manager to try to set standards across a whole range of professional work without advice from the particular professional group.

The third essential component of leadership is to be clear what the department's role is and to end up with each member of staff also being sure of what their individual jobs are within the overall role. Such clarity is a preconditon to being a productive and contributing member of the organization. Only then will the job they do fit into place and be seen to be purposeful. Equally such a well-understood state of affairs will significantly encourage initiatives and a broader contribution from staff. Such is the lesson of research [5] but even more is it self evident in terms of common sense. The more skilled and professional the workforce, the greater such understanding, and consequent commitment, should be.

Fourthly, delegation is fundamental to effective leadership. It is impossible for a manager to do the job properly if time is spent doing the work of subordinate staff. Managers at all levels fall into this trap, partly because it is easier to do work with which they may be very familiar; they may after all have been promoted directly from doing just this work. The manager may also be very apprehensive about letting go and doing the managerial job because he himself has not been trained or made to feel confident in it. Sometimes a manager will rationalize that it is quicker to do the job himself rather than show a subordinate how to do it. The response to this, of course, is apart from it not being the manager's job, that the subordinate will never be able to do a particular job unless allowed, encouraged and trained to do so.

The ability to delegate soundly is an important attribute of an effective leader as long as clarity of purpose and role is ensured, as well as making sure the subordinate staff are properly trained and are genuinely allowed to get on with the job. In doing so they will put more energy into it providing they agree what is to be done with their manager. Often they can then be left to work out for themselves, within reason, the way in which the work is done.

The leader's fifth essential role is to make sure subordinate staff have the tools to do the job in terms of environment, equipment and training and to make it possible for staff themselves to comment on the sorts of tools that are most useful. The armed services have been most keenly aware of the need for equipping staff to do the job to the highest possible standard and such lessons were most dramatically learned in the Second World War especially in the preparations for D-Day. Leaders and managers must understand that although bad workers may at times blame their tools no progress will be made even by a good worker unless the proper equipment is available. The leader will very quickly be seen as ineffectual and unsupportive of his subordinates if this essential is not met. If a team is to be built then the leader will be looked to, to press the case of the group as much as is practicable, consistent with the aims of the organization. The manager who expects support but does not give it will quickly be isolated.

Leadership through influence

In some senses the essence of leadership and, therefore, of management, is the constant conditioning and influencing of staff. Such processes conducted in a pejorative way would tend to be negative and create suspicion. Used constructively and openly, however, they are processes for positive benefit and are accepted by all concerned as worthwhile. The power of conditioning and influencing is very great. The effects of advertising and the media both for the good and bad effects they have are well recognized. Employees are susceptible to conditioning and influencing and managers must recognize and use this in a responsible way. Many managers influence staff without realizing that they are doing so. Every transaction that takes place between a manager and subordinate staff has an impact on all parties. Bad influencing causes resentment, confusion, a feeling of ill will and lack of commitment whereas beneficial influencing creates a continuum of clarity, understanding, awareness and commitment as well as a feeling of being important and useful through which staff feel confident about commenting on the organization and putting forward ideas for improvement.

In the health services, and amongst professionals in particular, full advantage of the good or quiet times is not taken. Such periods should be used for building the style and motivational foundations that give solid support in more turbulent times. To try to build participative or democratic styles of management during a turbulent phase is impossible, as many managers in all sectors of the labour market have discovered. If built in the quiet phases, however, and if built substantially, such a style will create trust and confidence which will usually carry an organization through bad times. The inherent individuality of health professionals suggests that an approach or management style that does not recognize such individuality will create tensions in a work group that can become destructive and time consuming. In positive terms if clarity of purpose is achieved and each member of staff is fully used and involved, the professional jealousies reduce to insignificance or constructive levels, a cohesion within the department is created and the manager sees himself not as the fount of knowledge or authority but more a *primus inter pares*, an initiator and co-ordinator.

REFERENCES

1. Mandy C. B. (1976) *Understanding Organization*, Penguin, Harmondsworth.
2. Maslow, A. M. (1954) *Motivation and Personality*, Harper & Row, New York.
3. McGregor, D. (1960) *The Human Side of Enterprise*, McGraw-Hill, New York.
4. Mayo, E. (1945) *The Social Problems of an Industrial Civilisation*, The

Andover Press, USA; Boston, Massachusetts. Roethlisberger, F. J. and Dickson, W. J. (1979) *Management and the Worker*, Harvard University Press. Cambridge, Massachusetts.
5. Humble, J. W. (1969) *Improving Management Performance*, British Institute of Management, London.

Chapter 5

Creating a productive working climate

The environment in which staff work has a number of components. Bearing in mind the complexity and variability of people, it is important that all the components that impinge on a person's productivity are considered and then made more conducive to improving that productivity. The working environment encompasses any physical, organizational or operational element, that has an impact on the work an employee does, the amount they do and the standard which they attain.

The main environmental factors that need to be considered fall into three main categories. There are those to do with the physical aspects of work (the buildings, equipment, lighting, physical safety). Then there are the psychological and intellectual aspects which are largely to do with how the business is structured organizationally and how its managers go about motivating and dealing with staff. Finally there are the emotional and the social aspects of the workplace, which we have already seen are important and there needs to be some outline of how improvements can be made to aid productivity.

THE PHYSICAL ELEMENTS

These elements have clear direct links back to Maslow's model about the hierarchy of needs and although it would be unproductive to squeeze each element into one of the levels, the model helps to get the various elements into a context. Unless employees' needs are met in a logical order, their motivation and productivity will be in jeopardy. Their manager is the person who has the authority and ability to get the working environment or climate right. To do so it is most logical to start with the physical elements.

Only change the changeable

Few managers can influence where a workplace is situated or what constitutes the main physical layout. Whilst such elements are important, if they can no longer be affected, then it is wise not to spend energy on them. It is much more practical to spend time changing those things that are changeable.

It is important primarily to get the basics right. Many managers still regard it as someone else's job to discover and put right leaks in roofs, draughty and cold rooms and dingy offices. If these matters are of concern to staff and affect their productivity, then it is the manager's responsibility to correct them. It may take time and effort but it is almost self-evident that someone's capacity for work will drop if rain water is leaking into the area where they work or even worse dripping from the ceiling. Such a scenario may seem to many to be somewhat extreme but experience shows that such episodes are commonplace especially in older hospitals.

The legal standards

With buildings, equipment and other priorities such as lighting and heating, the law has a role in setting certain standards. These, however, are concerned with basic level needs such as safety. Most of these laws[1] legislate on matters of safety, health and basic facilities at the workplace. In this context these are the Factories Acts (most recent of which is 1961), the Offices, Shops and Railway Premises Act, 1963, the Health and Safety at Work etc. Act, 1974 and the regulations that emanate from them.

The aim of these Acts is twofold, the first of which is to develop a statutory and administrative framework within which health and safety at work can be promoted. The second, although strongly linked to the first, is to specify certain things that must or must not be done in the direct interest of health and safety at work. The first aim is met largely by the 1974 Act and the second by most other legislation and regulations. A typical provision for a specific mandatory standard is that which requires a minimum temperature in certain premises – namely offices, shops and railway premises – where, under the 1963 Act, the temperature must have reached 16°C after the first hour of working. This Act, the Factories Act and the resultant regulations, are largely made up of lists of standards that must be met, which, over time, have become more comprehensive. It is a manager's job to know the constraints and conditions imposed on him by law and policy and whilst it is not practical to be aware of all the clauses that might be applicable, ignorance will often not be an excuse for omission. The Health and Safety at Work Act helps a great deal in this for it requires organizations to have an overall health and safety policy which will require each department to have a local policy. Such a policy will, or should, set out all the minimum standards that relate to the health and safety of all who use the department and will need to cover buildings, equipment and systems of work.

Effects of safety on productivity

There are naturally links between such standards and the productivity of staff. Some might argue that there are some precautions that might reduce productivity and in a sense they might be right. In the engineering trades, for example, there are many examples where employees, often encouraged by their managers, have not used machine guards, or have cut corners in other ways, to increase production. The safety consequences have often been dire with maiming injuries and even death being caused. Such a view cannot be justified on ethical, legal or even practical grounds as injuries cost industry a great deal in compensation and lost time. The most telling example in the health services is to do with back injuries[2] where in the average general hospital just over 20% of all reported accidents to staff are caused by bad or untimely lifting with injury being caused to the back. Some of these injuries resolve very quickly but others do not. The pain and discomfort they cause are difficult to measure and although the lost time is easier to analyse there is a great deal of hidden lost time caused by staff who have a back problem, either working slower than they might otherwise or merely taking annual rather than sick leave when the pain reaches a certain level. Additionally, there are those staff who have to leave their job because their injury is unlikely to resolve sufficiently. The number of professionals who leave for this reason is difficult to assess accurately because although some claim industrial injury benefit or early pensions it is probable that many do not and quietly and somewhat stoically leave. It would be very surprising if the figure were less than 500 per year from the professions allied to medicine (physiotherapy and nursing especially) within the NHS and the figure could be much higher; and this only from injured backs. Other injuries cause as much discomfort and affect productivity as seriously. It is clear, therefore, that the manager, especially of health professionals who set standards and example, should look to improve health and safety systems for humanitarian as well as purely economic reasons.

Even though most could recognize that there are strong positive links between safety and productivity, the standards laid down by law are not aimed at improving productivity. Improvements in the physical environment to do this are the employing organization's and manager's job, so what main areas should they concentrate on once the basic standards of shelter and safety have been met?

The layout and ambiance of the workplace

Of most impact on many staff is whether a department is attractive – at least in the sense that it is physically a reasonably welcoming place to come into and work within. To achieve such an atmosphere can be quite a cheap operation, it may only be a question of decoration or small adjustments to internal layout. Internal layout has rather more far-reaching implications, however, on the flow of work if components of a job are done by one person and then passed on to another for the next process. The obvious examples where layouts have major impacts on workflow, apart from hospital ward areas, are departments such as outpatient departments and process departments like radiography, pharmacy and pathology laboratories. Many such departments expand a little like Topsy with little overall plan, except when moving into a new building. A manager would be well advised to regularly review the layout of a department in the context of the work processes and amenability, both of which often complement each other. It is useful to try metaphorically to view the department from a height and from the sides so the total process can be seen. If a review in depth is felt necessary, it may be best to call in help from a work-study engineer who will be expert in work flows and time and motion study and will have a knowledge of areas of good practice as well as the pitfalls to be avoided.

Temperature and air

Health services managers and staff are often preoccupied by the warmth or chilliness of the departments they work in. Leaving aside the element to do with patient comfort and the standards accepted for employees (16°C is not very warm for a sedentary worker), it is important to consider heating but not in isolation. Humidity and whether air is fresh or stagnant also have significant effects on work rates and the combination of any two or three is crucial. The New York Ventilation Commission [3], whose work has been confirmed time and again since then, showed as early as 1923, that for fairly physically active work (the sort of work many professional health workers are involved in) that output depended on certain features; 20°C, was found to be the most efficacious temperature as long as air was fresh. Changes in temperature and air have significant effects. Such changes illustrated in Table 5.1 are very common in most workplaces and very much greater ones are well known in hospital departments.

When overly dry or humid conditions are superimposed on these figures they swing more violently. In particular high humidity of more than 80% causes particular drops in output, especially where physical work is involved, so those who have influence over heating and air conditioning systems need to take note of the balances needed. The individual manager can do a number of things to bring about the best balance. A specification can be laid down, appropriate to the sort of work done in a department, for the engineer responsible for heating and ventilation. Where this does not work or some fine tuning is needed, judicious manipulation of radiator values and opening or closing of windows or doors can bring about improvements in temperature, humidity and movement of air.

Table 5.1 Effects of temperature and air movement on physical work

Temperature (°C)	Air	Units of Work (100 = optimum)	Fall in output due to stagnant air	Fall in output due to rise in temperature	Total fall in output
20°	Fresh	100.0			
20°	Stagnant	91.1	8.9		8.9
24°	Fresh	85.2		14.8	14.8
24°	Stagnant	76.2	8.6	15.2	23.8

Every winter there is exhortation to keep windows closed when heating is on to save energy. If, however, the resultant climate is hot, stagnant and very dry, work output may drop, in some cases by 40–50% so not only is there a balance to be struck between temperature, air movement and humidity but between costs of heating and benefits to work output.

Effects of lighting

There is now much advice on type and intensity of lighting and their effects on eyesight, headaches and to a lesser extent on productivity. The rapid growth in the use and number of visual display units, for example, has heightened the awareness of lighting[4]. However, work done before this growth indicated the importance of what can best be described as lighting that is comfortable for the work that is performed. General diffused light is all that is necessary in some areas of an organization, such as dining or coffee lounges. Four times the intensity of light is needed for precision work needing a high level of definition and concentration than for reading a good print of the average typewriter size[5]. Good lighting can be cheerful and stimulating and so is capable of improving morale.

Rarely, do people comment favourably about strip or fluorescent lighting, usually because it normally has a marked flicker and often has a very white, almost blue white light. Both of these phenomena are unnatural and invariably people prefer light that has a daylight colour – which is also the most effective visually.

Basic ergonomic considerations

If the manager is concerned about the comfort and consequent morale and productivity of staff, much consideration must also be given to individual staff's physical requirements. Many sedentary workers could talk at great length about the discomfort they go through after long periods of sitting in badly designed chairs at equally badly designed desks working with ergonomically inefficient machines. Major improvements have been made in ergonomic knowledge and the design of furniture and equipment but still public organizations particularly tend to buy what is initially cheap equipment but which may be, in the long run, very inefficient or even injurious, especially to backs. Equally, much equipment designed to be used by non-sedentary workers is designed to be efficient in what it does but, until recently, with little thought given to designing it so that it fits naturally to the person who is going to use it time and again. Equipment that makes the operator bend frequently, stretch beyond comfortable limits, twist or lean are all to be avoided.

The most effective way to ensure that appropriate equipment is installed, or revamped so it is made more amenable, is to take advice on specific equipment and its application from trained ergonomists especially where the equipment is going to feature significantly in the staff's working day. Equally useful is to consult in detail with the staff who are going to use the equipment. Not only will they be able to outline most, if not all, the potential trouble spots and causes of discomfort and inefficiency, but having been involved in the decision on choice, will feel much more involved and committed. It is somewhat incongruous for the manager who is not going to use a piece of equipment, to choose it and for someone who is going to use it every day not to be involved in that choice. The incongruity increases when a group with no links to the particular department chooses the equipment in isolation, as can happen with supplies or procurement departments which do not involve users. The most propitious process is probably for the manager to decide on the basic specification, which would include some ergonomic elements and then within some constraints, such as finance, leave the ultimate choice to the user.

Rate of work

Whilst not part of the physical fabric of a building, many of the requirements of the job itself contribute to, or detract from, the productiveness of the overall physical environment. The rate at which people are expected to work can have a major effect on total output. Motor manufacturers learned the hard way that unless laid-down work rates were seen as practicable and fair then output targets could not be met. Not only would such targets not be achieved but other, often long-term, industrial relations problems would be likely to arise.[6] Although not suggesting that tortoiselike work intensities should be the aim, the tortoise was the one who achieved his goal. Similarly it can be quite salutary to watch experienced manual crafts people or labourers at work. They give an impression of not being at all frenetic but work steadily to a rhythm and produce much more by the end of the working day. There is a British Standard that is used as a baseline for bonus and productivity schemes which recognizes this fact in that a work rate of about 70% of capacity is the most effective long-term rate. The manager of a department should take advantage of such experience for not only will output or productivity benefit and fatigue (and possibly consequent accidents) be kept down, but also feelings about a fair day's pay for a fair day's work will evolve. Morale will consequently improve and a virtuous and productive circle be created.

There is no intrinsic virtue in work, despite the puritan and Victorian ethics that suggest otherwise. The value of work comes from what it produces, be that a manufactured product or a service or merely a sense of achievement or satisfaction. Nor is there practical benefit in driving staff so hard that they become exhausted and disenamoured with what they are doing or even why they are doing it. Such activity may give the appearance of being busy and so being productive but usually such is not the case.

Where efficiency, safety, health and morale are of significant concern equipment can often be used to help or even take over some of the more laborious functions that people have had to do in the past. Consideration will need to take account of costs, benefits as well as the feelings and traditions of staff. Technology is advancing so rapidly that many managers become bemused at the range of equipment increasingly becoming available to the health professions.

Although some equipment is out of date by the time it is installed the manager needs to consider the purpose of a piece of equipment and judge whether it helps staff do their job better and more safely now and for the expected life of the equipment. It is seductive but usually unhelpful to put off buying a machine today because there might be a deluxe and more sophisticated version round the corner. The deluxe version may do additional things but such things may not be useful to the particular department and by procrastinating no progress at all is made.

ORGANIZATION AND COMMUNICATIONS SYSTEMS

The physical environment is clearly of great significance in the productivity and morale of an organization. It is, however, only part of the story. The organizational aspects are as crucial but more dynamic, more susceptible to misinterpretation and often less tangible. These are matters that are strongly affected by, and in turn influence the organizational structure, how people are managed, how they are regarded and communicated with, some of which have already been discussed. They are also concerned with the need to develop morale, manage the tension and stresses in the organization and turn them into forces for, and not against, productivity and quality.

The need for structure

The organizational structure of a business or a hospital is the cornerstone of managing. The principles and methods of organizational design are discussed in the next chapter but the need for a defined order or framework is important for a number of reasons. The prime reason is that each of the component parts of an organization need to be defined in terms of its shape, size and nature and also their position, role and authority relative to all the others. The way of looking at a job in the context of its demands, choices and constraints has already been discussed at some length (see Chapter 2). Unless these are clear in an individual job definition and, more generally, unless the way jobs relate with each other so that duplication and overlap are kept to an absolute minimum, the framework within which people work will become confusing. The main essence of a structure in management or organizational terms is that it lays out an understood and logical framework within which effective work is done. As an integral part of this the demands, choices and constraints are clarified. Although organizational structures are not the reason for an organization existing, a good one will positively promote a productive working environment, a poor one will hold progress and productivity back.

Objectives of restructuring

There are a number of problems that many managers may create when reviewing their structures. First, they tend to try to squeeze the organization of a department or a larger unit of management into a preconceived or prescribed form that fits with some good theory but fails to take account of past history, culture and attitudes. Secondly, restructuring is seen as an end in itself rather than a mechanism through which progress is helped and promoted. Often a manager will restructure a department and then sit back waiting for results. Such action is rather like designing and making a new tool but not picking it up and actively using it. Thirdly and most frequently, new structures, and often new systems, are superimposed on preexisting ones with very little review, change or discarding of the old. The end result is something of a hybrid or even a series of structural or systems strata laid on top of each other which prevents either the new or the old working well. A proper review would spend as much time dismantling the old as building the new and making sure all concerned know about both facets.

If clarity is the essence of any structure, simplicity should be the theme. If a structure becomes complex it loses the ability to promote many of the key management processes, most significantly of all the communications. Communication in a large organization can become complex merely because of size and it takes consciousness and determination to maintain simplicity and promote good communications.

Communications and the structure

Communications is not a process set apart from management responsibility. Too often faults or mistakes that take place in a business, and frequently in health services, are put down to a breakdown in communications. Such may be the immediate cause of the problem but the root cause will be management ineptness or failure somewhere along the line. It somehow sounds excusable to blame a breakdown in communications rather than managerial negligence, forgetfulness or incompetence. It also makes it harder to pinpoint responsibility. Communications systems are inert mechanisms – they neither succeed not fail. The people who use them determine the success of communications within an organization, although the tools they use can be sharpened or made more relevant to the task in hand.

Communications guidelines

The importance of communications is, however, not questioned. Without it no employee will know what to do or why, nor will there be adequate feedback to the higher levels of the organization. The significance of joint involvement in the business of the organization has been discussed; the criteria for communicating, the ways of doing it and its benefits are not so apparent.

The basic criterion that should govern any process of communications is the need to know. Such a need may be created by the technical content of a job and someone has to be told to cope with certain elements of the job or some sanction will be imposed. A different need may exist because it is important to keep staff in touch with some issue, not because it is an integral part of their job but because it paints a wider picture of a general work-related interest and by keeping people in touch they become more committed to the whole enterprise, and understand where they fit into it. The need for the manager to be seen as a focal point will be promoted if he is seen as a timely and trustworthy communicator. Frequently much information gets to staff by systems other than the line management structure. The local press, trade unions and often other staff are the usual pre-emptive sources.

Conditioning and influencing

Communications may be used to influence or condition people in the organization systematically or on an *ad hoc* basis. Many large companies conduct corporate style advertising rather than particular product advertising to get an image about the company across to the public and also very specifically to employees. Companies that have developed policies concerning quality promotion or that emphasize putting the customer first, advertise very largely to create a self-fulfilling ambiance for the employees who are expected to deliver the improved standards implied by the advertising.

There may also be a need to communicate merely to keep part of the organization or an external body informed, just to keep it from interfering in the local or internal processes or merely to generate kudos in being involved.

Communication should not just be from the top down. Communication of information, ideas, worries, delight, anger, comment and so on is a multidirectional process and continuous. The manager has as much responsibility to listen actively as to talk to subordinate staff and colleagues on the same level. Similarly a profession or a health authority has a responsibility to listen to staff, consumers and colleagues from other professions. Such communications if pursued diligently promote a dynamic system within which employees at all levels feel at ease, well informed and committed. The essential result of any communications is that something is done with the information, idea or comment communicated and that some positive result ensues.

Overcommunicating

Although the more junior levels of staff tend to feel they never get the whole picture, it is possible to overcommunicate. The most frequent examples for managers in the health services are being inundated with memoranda or circulars cascading from the top of the organization to the bottom with intervening levels of management often only pausing to put a circulation list on the top and sending them on down the line. Such a blanket approach can be dangerous as it may not be clear who should take necessary action and often because a memorandum lands on someone's desk they may assume they need take no action as the memorandum has gone to many others and in any case there is no specific instruction for them. What the intervening levels of management should do is to consider and decide what needs to be done with such missives and then send it on only with comment or instruction. The question 'who needs to know, why and how?' needs to be answered each time.

Using communications to shift responsibility

Managerially, in terms of responsibility and authority, an equally common and dangerous form of communications in the health services is the inferred delegation upwards. This occurs when a member of staff or manager suggests to their manager they are communicating a piece of information or a comment merely to keep them informed. Frequently the real reason will be to avoid responsibility for taking action or not as the case may be. Unless the transaction between the two is very clear, that it is or is not delegation of responsibility one way or the other, grave confusion can ensue. Such confusion will enable the more junior manager to protest, if the issue goes awry, that he told his senior and so the responsibility was passed upwards. The more senior manager's responsibility in such circumstances is to make it quite clear where the responsibility rests and in doing so has completed the communication which may at the outset have been unnecessary. It becomes clear, therefore, that the most effective structural line of communications is the management line which is synonymous with the lines of accountability and delegation. Going outside these lines will, again, create confusion especially amongst those being communicated with.

Methods of communicating

Having established the principles of communication, some of the more useful methods become germane. All forms of communication have some distortion in them. If the simplest form of communication is between two individuals the message can be distorted by the way it is put by the sender [7]. This is because of the language he uses has shades of meanings to him, and has certain values and biases, particularly if the message is a spoken one and it is very susceptible to nuance and tone. Secondly the receiver has understandings of language values and philosophy. The third place where distortion and misunderstanding take place is in the process of communication itself or in the medium. In practice the process is made complex by the matrix of different lines of communication, the different levels at which it takes place, whether it is formal or informal, or the medium that is used. There is some hope, however, in that in the practical setting there is usually the chance for feedback, response, correction, reinforcement or confirmation. Any form of communication in the personnel management context should allow for each of these elements to be used fully enough for the right and intended message to get through. There have been a number of systems designed to create clarity and speed of communications at work, the best known of which is the concept of Team Briefing devised by the Industrial Society.

Forms of communication

Communications are verbal, both written and oral, and non-verbal, predominantly the use of, and reaction to, body language [8]. People can also communicate notions or images through how they dress and present themselves.

People adopt a much more permissive cultural attitude to such matters as dress, but most are still very much influenced by it. The obvious example for the health professions is what a uniform means to colleagues and patients. It confers a certain status on he who wears it so he will be taken more or less seriously depending on what the uniform denotes – profession, rank or status – as well as how it is worn, smartly or slovenly.

Although non-verbal forms of communication are significant the use of words and language in a business setting is the most important.

Verbal communications
The main components in verbal communication other than the distorting components such as bias, assumptions, stereotyping, understanding of language used, values and double meanings

are the process and medium used. In getting the message over it is important not to assume that the receiver knows too much about the subject under discussion. Almost certainly the sender and receiver will start from different points of understanding so the first thing to do is to give an outline of what is under discussion, set the limits and definitions and, if it helps, give some background information. This is in effect setting the agenda. Then it will help if a response is sought to check a common position. If two parties start off from different positions but each believes he understands the other's the degree of error or divergence not only gets built into the process but usually widens and misunderstandings increase.

Such a process is important in all oral and most written communications whether it be on a one-to-one basis or in a large group. Whilst some of the dynamics of groups may be different from those present in one-to-one transactions the fundamental processes are similar. Most business communication – oral or written – has an element of negotiated order about it which will mean that the process of communicating, once the start point is agreed will be one of proposition and response, defining and clarifying and as long as the genuine opportunity is given for feedback, correction, reinforcement and comment then the clearer and more defined the communication will be.

The virtue of written communications is that it represents a physical record of what is communicated. However, the written word is as capable of interpretation as the spoken one and therein lies the main disadvantage of written communications when sloppily expressed. Written communications take on a more formal, established or authoritative status merely because they are written which means that particular care is needed in their composition. The added danger is that written communications are on the record and may be used and misinterpreted in the future when memories about the real reason for, and nuances behind, the communication are dim. If such a likelihood is probable (it is always possible) then an unambiguous interpretation must be contained in the document.

Meetings
In terms of creating a positive working climate the spoken word is, in transactions with staff, almost always the more effective as long as time is devoted to it.

The one-to-one meeting is the basic form. Whether or not this is formal, that is prearranged, with a set purpose, or informal such as a chance meeting in a corridor or at lunch, the big advantage is that both parties can propose, respond, give information, clarify and go through all the processes without being diverted by others. Proportionately more time by far is given to an individual in this forum than in a large meeting, so with all these characteristics, the outcome should be unambiguous. A disadvantage is that unless the discussion has taken place between the only two people who need to know, or be involved, then the whole process must be gone through again at least once and if outcomes are different, that in itself will pose a problem.

Such disadvantages can be overcome with a larger meeting of say three or four to eight or nine in number. Such meetings also have the virtue of getting a number of minds applied to a problem which can often be productive and also get the commitment of all concerned to a particular course of action. A disadvantage is that the depth of discussion is often limited because whoever is running the meeting feels constrained by time and the need to let everyone who wants to contribute to do so. Some employees are often reluctant to speak up in meetings of any sort involving more than four or five people, especially when they are junior amongst a number of more senior and experienced professionals. When this happens a useful contribution may be lost and a member of staff feel undervalued or disgruntled. The reverse side of this particular coin is that there may be a speaker who holds the floor more to demonstrate how important he is than to make a positive contribution. The chairman will need to strike a balance in both circumstances.

The larger meeting still, for example a staff meeting or mass departmental meeting, is best designed for the transmission of information rather than the discussion of and decision on issues. Large meetings used in any other way than for passing information and clarifying what the information means, are difficult to handle and it is too easy to assume that certain courses of action are agreed at them, when in fact no such agreement is achieved. The main reasons for this lie in the intrinsic difficulties of communication, namely it is impractical to expect to get a common understanding, unity of interpretation and a common basis for any apparent agreement on an issue which by definition, will contain some conflict of interest. It may be more effective to run a series of smaller meetings and gain progressive agreement on the issue. Such agreement needs to be progressive in most instances as otherwise significant progress with one group may be put back by disagreement with another. A more effective way of communicating information and of strengthening the commitment to the particular management structure, is to charge each level of management to communicate to a pattern through a system of team briefing. The pattern will depend upon the brief that each manager has been given and will ensure the consistency of the message.

Negotiation, where there is a significant conflict of interest, as often exemplified by management/trade union negotiations, is a form of communication that has many of the usual characteristics, so should not cause too much worry to managers. Often, however, the issue is substantial or there is a lot of tension generated because of the ritualistic stances taken up by both sides – something many professional health workers are even now not used to. These differences and ways of coping with them will be discussed in Chapter 7.

The telephone
Communications by telephone should not be regarded as any different to one-to-one oral communications, except that the non-verbal responses and signals, other than silence, are not available. This means that the participants need to be more careful about interpretation and what is really being said. Otherwise if there is any doubt, or even room for doubt, it would be advisable to meet or to summarize and clarify until there is certainty of message. This is one of the reasons why written confirmation of the result of a telephone call is often asked for and is often a sensible feature. As electronic aids to communication, such as networked personal computers and conference and facsimile systems, become more common such confirmation of, and clarity in, communication will become much more practicable.

The emphasis given to effective communications is intentional. Without it confusion and aimlessness quickly take over; with it a sense of direction, clarity of purpose, a sense of belonging and morale all improve. It is the key tool at the disposal of the manager who consequently needs to keep it well honed.

Security within the organization

Most people, and especially those who have the vocation to join one of the various health professions, generally say they need a solid base with a feeling of security. If an employee is constantly apprehensive about future employment, his commitment to the job, especially in the medium and long term, will be low and consequently his energy and productivity correspondingly so.

Fixed-term and rolling contracts
With the inception of the philosophy of general management [9] into the national health service, came the policy that senior managers would be employed on fixed-term contracts of employment of three or five years or on rolling contracts. Whilst it can be argued with some justification that the attitude engendered by being subject to a fixed-term contract may sharpen the mind and encourage performance, the type of performance that is encouraged tends to be concerned with short-term goals. In addition, the very fact that the contract has a fixed term, fixes the mind of the holder on the end of the term, making him not only concentrate on short-term issues but become very uncertain about his future. Coping with so much apprehension can easily become counterproductive to the real job in hand.

General job insecurity
Extreme effects of insecurity are observed when a work group is informed that a department or hospital may be closing down or moving particularly when there is high unemployment in the area. Morale drops, those who can find other work do so, leaving behind them a further demoralized set whose productivity drops and the members of which frequently consider industrial action; not with any real hope of reversing a decision to close but more as the only expression of anger, frustration or helplessness that they can make. Such examples have been infrequent in the health services, but are becoming more common. Usually, however, health authorities are big enough to absorb any staff shaken out by a small hospital closing, at least so far as professional groups are concerned.

Professional security
By and large, however, most health services offer their professional staff groups considerable and real job security which

enables most staff to have no major concerns over future employment. Feelings of insecurity do arise as times of organizational tension as recent (1982 and 1984) reorganizations have illustrated. Frequently, such tensions are created more by worries about what the status of a particular profession or the promotion or career prospects of individuals and groups are likely to be in the future and as is usually the case, such worries are based on the unknown rather than hard facts. The only way in which such tensions can be dealt with are by ensuring future plans and structure are as well known as possible and that individuals are handled with sensitivity.

The form of security that, by experience, most staff work best within is to know that on balance their job is safe as long as they perform reasonably and that they are going to be managed in a consistent and even-handed way. If they have this then the climate in which they do their job will enable them to get on with it positively. Amongst professionals especially this has to be balanced by a willingness to change and keep up to date with new techniques, technologies and clinical standards.

STRESS IN THE WORKPLACE

Tension, and to some extent stress, can be positive forces and no organization could operate effectively, or at all, without them. Athletes, actors, public speakers and ordinary staff all perform or work better if their minds are sharpened or 'psyched up', on a particular matter. They become a negative force when they exist in such amounts or in such a form that they have a demoralizing and even an alienating effect on groups and individuals, even to the extent of causing mental and physical illness. A common manifestation is not necessarily real illness, in the clinical sense, but a propensity to give in to trivial complaints and stay away from work because there is little commitment to do otherwise.

A significant potential for stress exists in the interface between home and work and this needs to be recognized in the work organization and management style. It is already recognized that workers are 'twenty-four hour' people in that their domestic values and pressures affect them at work and vice versa. Most employees take their concerns about work home and bring domestic worries to work. Often pressure from one area exacerbates problems in the other. This becomes especially true when workload is high or deadlines are approaching at work or when there are domestic problems or illness at home. The manager must recognize such stress creation elements and whilst it may not be possible to resolve the root cause, especially if it lies in the domestic camp, account can be taken of the pressures a member of staff may be going through and give time, help and space to help the individual work through the difficulties. To suggest that the individual should not bring home-problems to work is impractical and negative in that it will not help resolve the domestic problems or their effects on work.

Analysts have become more aware of the amount of stress and its effects. They are in little doubt that it has increased in real and apparent terms [10]. The reasons are not difficult to discern: pressure to increase workload, little or no real control of workload, the increased pace of life generally and work-related issues particularly, increased possibilities of litigation or complaint especially against professional clinical workers and increased pressure to progress one's career. The organization and the managers within it should be able to manage many of these pressures and their resultant stress and reduce them to a manageable and even constructive level.

Reducing stress by planning

Ways in which this can be done are by planning the workload of a department and as objectively as possible matching staffing and skill levels to workload. It is recognized this is not easy especially as the pressures to increase output come from many different groups such as patients, doctors, senior managers and employing authorities as well as from the very nature of the work professionals do. It may be a stressful experience to know that one is not giving an adequate service to all those who need it and the frustration of many perceived constraints, such as financial resources and skilled staff, exacerbate this. The vicious circle has started. The manager, through planning priorities, not only gets more understood order into the work of a professional department but also takes a substantial share of the responsibility for what is done and, more importantly, what has to be left undone. The standard and quality of work done is now seen as much more controllable than in the past. Many health professions are already planning to set standards of quality on the work that is done. This adds a dimension to the quantity dealt with. A balanced amalgam of quantity and quality gives a firm basis on which to organize the work, plan or bid for additional resources or to make objective decisions on what work should not be done. Such objectivity has the virtues of helping to determine priorities and once determined reduce feelings of guilt that are otherwise caused by work being undone. Through this sort of planning and the work scheduling that flows from it, the organization and even the community at large begin to appreciate, and accept much more readily, the fact that not all the work needed can be done.

Management of work to reduce stress

Another tool the manager has, if stress is being caused by a peak of workload, is to smooth the peak out either by drafting extra staff or other resources in; usually difficult but not impossible if a bank or register of skilled labour is maintained. Many trained professionals do not want to work on a permanent or full-time basis but are willing to work on a casual basis when opportunities arise. Such banks and registers are used by some professional groups, nursing being the biggest example, but every staff group has a similar potential. The other ways of handling a peak of work are to either decide consciously and logically that some of it is not going to be done or, usually more acceptable, decide to extend the time over which it is done. This fourth dimension of time is the most under-managed by most people, managers of staff especially.

Ignorance-induced stress

Much stress is created by frustration, which, in turn, is caused by staff not knowing what is going on, feeling unable to influence their part of the organization in a way they feel well able to. They may also feel they are being undervalued, feeling threatened in job or professional terms and undergoing or being subject to change that they do not understand or are not committed to.

Most of these causes can be controlled by the manager, mainly by sensitive and timely communications, that is keeping staff fully informed and involved. It also means that the contribution that staff make needs to be regularly acknowledged. Too often if managers acknowledge the work of a member of staff it has been to do with a special or *ad hoc* piece of work whereas the value staff have, and that should be recognized, is the routine work and contribution they make day in, day out. Recognition of this can be during regular meetings or by making a special effort to acknowledge it at certain times such as during an appraisal session or when planning the next few months work. The real killer is indifference as it is in any relationship, and at work indifference by a manager for what staff do and feel amounts to managerial incompetence – it is after all the manager's prime job to manage and motivate the staff accountable to him.

Manifestations of stress

Stress, when it becomes unbearable, can manifest itself in conflict especially where a group of staff is involved in groups and Chapter 7 addresses the issue of resolving such conflict or differences. With individuals, however, one of its more advanced results is real illness, mental, physical or a combination of the two. No general prescription can be given for what is a very individual problem other than to advise that the last thing a sufferer needs is to be told to pull himself together. Stress-related illness should be handled in part like any other sickness but also it is important to find out the root causes so something can be done. In organizations where morale is reckoned to be low, absenteeism and stress-related illness are often high. Whilst it is right to help the individual through counselling and other support systems, it is also crucial to review why stress is being created and to reduce it to constructive proportions.

Building in fairness and other values

If the organization is not seen to be even handed and fair, the organizational climate may deteriorate and become unproductive. Most of all the fairness of the organization will be judged by the way in which staff are treated, how they are recruited, trained, dealt with when subject to discipline, promoted and handled when sick short term or suffer long-term ill health. Fairness does not necessarily mean that each person is treated in a way that is liked; more it suggests that staff know where they stand, are not singled out for special treatment or victimization, and are treated consistently with other staff and in line with the understood ethics and policies of the organization.

Other than being made to feel a genuine part of the organization, one of the most significant indicators of a good working climate is how staff feel they will be handled or treated when they are stressed or ill. Most of the values an organization has, impinge on the way in which an individual is treated in such circumstances. Is he valued, does he know what is going to happen, is he kept in touch, is he treated according to stated guidelines and policies, are his rights recognized and protected, is he treated as others are and are all the circumstances of any misfortune taken into account? The circumstances and points at issue can obviously vary greatly.

Handling absence – as an exercise in consistency

A manager will generally no doubt deal more robustly with the person who is absent every Monday and who it can be shown is swinging the lead or absent through self-inflicted abuse than the long-serving member of staff who has suffered a back injury at work and may be unable to return to work. Even in the first case all may not be as it appears and no management action should be taken unless by investigation all the relevant facts are known. The basic processes that need to be followed to ensure fairness and thus to promote an amenable climate, are to act as soon as concern about an individual occurs. Such concern may exist because of the nature of the illness, the pattern of attendance or the extra burden it is putting on colleagues. Then there is a need to enquire into all the facts and get the best advice necessary, both medical and personal, always keeping in close touch with the individual. Once this is done it is possible to consider a whole range of options, ranging from doing nothing, through developing a rehabilitation programme and counselling transfer to an easier job, to dismissal or retirement on the grounds of ill health or incapacity. Help is usually available on the detailed handling of all personnel problems. What the manager must do if an equable and productive climate is to be maintained is to act sooner rather than later, act consistently whilst considering the unique features of any problems and keep in very close touch with individuals involved.

Organizing for better morale

A great deal of implied and express mention of morale has been made in this chapter and the term deserves some attention. Often reference to morale is made by any level in the organization to express a feeling about 'them', 'them' being the levels above those making the comments. In effect, the term is used in stating that morale is high or low to suggest that something is right or wrong about the organization. Too frequently those who make such statements do not, or cannot, explain why they are suggesting a particular state of morale. It is often seen as rather fashionable, but irresponsible to say morale is the worst it has ever been with no obligation to account for such a statement. Nevertheless, the state of morale is crucial to the climate of the organization, in fact it is part of the climate. In outline, morale is to do with the level of confidence staff have in the organization as a whole or their part of it in particular. It can vary with time or with the part of the organization under scrutiny. The morale of a specific department may be very high yet across a hospital or the service as a whole or within a profession, morale may be seen as low. Too often morale is seen as synonymous with the levels of frustration in an organization. Such a straightforward conclusion has some validity but it does not go far enough. Frustrations and similar tensions exist in all organizations especially where employees are encouraged to use imagination and initiative. It is much more the ability of staff to resist those frustrations or the tensions that they give rise to that denotes the level and nature of morale. This being so it gives the guidance on how to measure the state of morale and consequently what to do about it.

The first apparent signs of lowering morale may well be bickering that is not directed at any particular issue but at the organization in general – often 'them'. Such is not always a bad sign; some degree of unsubstantiated criticism is a human trait, much as gossiping is; it is when it becomes counter-productive and self-perpetuating that the signs should be taken seriously. If they are not and morale dips further, open conflict can erupt but more dangerous is when the surface goes calm but underneath the bickering continues and progressively turns into conspiring. Individuals may well through their decreasing ability to resist frustration, behave in a number of ways. Assembly-line workers have been known to sabotage work sometimes in a trivial way but at other times in ways that are dangerous as has happened on car assembly lines in the USA and this country with brake lines not being connected and wheel nuts not being tightened when morale reached such low levels that employees were minded to vent their frustrations on or act defiantly against the company and even in extreme cases society at large [11]. Others may merely act more and more passively, not seeing themselves as being valued or of use and withdraw into a shell. They may do their job, just adequately or hide the inadequacies so that they are not discernible or do not come to light for some time. Such action, by both individuals and groups, often evolves into quite active refusals to co-operate so the manager's job becomes more difficult and output drops. In the health professions, the most common manifestations of low morale, apart from general bickering, are labour turnover.

Professional staff are normally a very marketable commodity and can practise their profession almost anywhere in the public or private sector or often on their own. If the climate at work created by the manager is such that the frustrations and tensions cannot be resisted then staff will leave. It may be that turnover is high for other reasons such as pay, although this can itself be an influence on morale. The important factor is, however, to recognize the signs and analyse the real causes either as a special management project or as part of the human resource planning process outlined in Chapter 3. Once that is done it is essential to take positive and substantial action. Low or high morale tend to be self-generating and self-fulfilling so if morale is low it needs special effort to turn it round. Once it is turned round, whilst it still needs to be worked at, it will tend to generate its own momentum.

It is important to recognize that morale is largely a state of attitude of mind based on factors that are substantially in the control of the manager. Again it is often indifference and insensitivity that lower it; involvement, communications, fairness and concern that raise it. Morale is one of the components, as well as one of the measures, that make up the overall climate of the organization; without giving it routine consideration, the climate will degenerate.

This climate is often alluded to when employers discuss aims such as the creation of good industrial relations. Such a phrase is woolly and can mean almost anything, depending on the person using it and the person or group about whom it is used. It is more constructive to address issues to do with improving the productiveness of the working climate, the efficacy of certain management style or the way in which an employer wishes to regard and develop the work force than to make bland value statements of vague aim. Managers need to concentrate on achieving a sense of direction, a clarity of purpose and role, stated aims and an actively pursued management culture in the organization. Such aims are capable of detailed definition, explanation and measurement. They are also clearly recognized when seen and only if these qualities are extant can any productive climate or environment be improved.

REFERENCES

1. Factories Act, 1961; Offices, Shops and Railway Premises Act, 1963; Health and Safety at Work etc. Act, 1974.
2. Ergonomics Research Unit (1984) *Back Pain in Nurses*, Robens Institute of Industrial and Environmental Health and Safety, University of Surrey.
3. *Report of the New York State Commission on Ventilation* (1923) E. P. Dutton (ed.), New York.
4. Institute of Personnel Management (1983) *People and VDUs*, IPM, London.
5. Tinker, M. A. (1947) Illumination Standards for Effective and Easy Seeing, *US Psychology Bulletin*, **44**, 435–450.
6. Beynon, H. (1973) *Working for Ford*, Penguin, Harmondsworth.
7. Argyle, M. and Trower, P. (1979) *Person to Person*, Harper & Row, London.

8. Morris, D. (1979) *Man Watching*, A field guide to Human behaviour, Abrams, New York.
9. *NHS Management Enquiry*. Letter to Secretary of State for Social Services from R. Griffiths (leader of enquiry) 1983. (Griffiths Report).
10. Smith, M., Beck, J., Cooper, C. L. *et al.* (1982) *Introducing Organisational Behavior*, ch.5. Macmillan, Basingstoke.
11. Beynon, H. (1973) *Working for Ford*, Penguin, Harmondsworth.

Part Three

Management in the Organization

Chapter 6

Organization design and staff development

Recruiting good staff into well-defined jobs creates a firm foundation, but much remains to be built upon this. The management of staff in any profession, but especially in those that are developing rapidly, needs to be viewed as a dynamic continuum. This is partly a factor of the health business, partly the organic nature of the health professions, rapidly changing techniques and technology and also due to the fact that constant change is part of the human condition. Having the right staff in the right jobs and yet recognizing that change is a permanent feature of managerial life, managers need to adjust the organizational structure and develop individual managers and staff within it to keep pace. An aim should be to control change rather than merely respond to it.

ORGANIZATION REVIEW AND CHANGE

Any change in design of structure or any plan to develop staff must flow in a logical sequence. The guiding light must be the mission or overall purpose of the organization and the way it proposes to achieve these. Then the structure needs to be developed in order to actively promote and achieve the aims. Such development needs to take account of the main tenets of effective organizational design. Having then prescribed the roles of individual jobs the next task is to develop the people in those jobs. This individual development is a managerial task that most managers recognize as a good thing but too few give the time, sustained effort and systematic attention that is needed and which gives a significant return on the investment.

Clarity of purpose

The first job in reviewing an organization is to be clear on its purpose or mission. Words like mission may have a rather evangelical connotation but when the word was first used in the late 1970s in respect of business organizations, it was recognized that the whole workforce, but most of all the managers, need to be enthusiastically committed to what the organization is in business for. It was also understood that those who are zealous in their commitment would put much more into the organization. The fundamental issue is, however, to be clear about the mission or purpose [1]. Over the past few years senior health managers have addressed such problems with much thought. Any statement on the purpose of a health authority, hospital or department must not be woolly or vague. Rather it must be concise and point to the way more detailed components of the organization will be designed. Such a statement should be the umbrella under which all objectives and aims are formed. Such a statement may include a comment or strong suggestion as to what the overall philosophy or style of the organization will be. An example might be that: 'this district (or hospital or department) is here to improve the health of the community by providing a range of high quality community and hospital-based care and treatment to meet the needs of individual consumers'.

Such a statement suggests that the organization must address health rather than just illness, that it owes a responsibility to the community it is situated in, that quality is an aim, and that the individuality of patients or consumers (denoting a consumer-orientated approach) is to be respected. Other elements could be added, for example to do with research, training and attitudes to staff. What is put in is the choice of the policy makers. A whole series of subphilosophies and aims or objectives will then flow from the prime purpose statement which will affect the way the organization is structured. If it is an aim to recognize that staff are a major asset and must be encouraged to develop their full potential, then a structure and jobs must be designed to ensure involvement of staff and to make sure adequate training and learning opportunities exist. It follows that job descriptions that do not emphasize the responsibilities of managers to appraise and train staff or a structure that does not have parts of it that promote training will not be compatible with the stated aim.

At the higher levels, such aims and purpose statements are not easy to frame without sounding trite. A way to avoid triteness or superficiality and the lack of commitment that goes with it, is to ensure that such statements contain strong pointers to subsidiary aims and objectives, that they are measurable and that once formulated the purpose and aims are not optional. Lower in the organization at hospital or department level it becomes easier to state purpose, aims and targets in that it is easier to be specific and quantitative. In professional departments, however, the very specificity can create problems in that the aims of the department may be different or in conflict with the aims of the professional that works in it. Such differences need to be reconciled or recognized in the aims statement and then in the structure that is designed. It would be a short-sighted statement at this level that did not recognize the particular professional features, such as a certain degree of clinical freedom *vis-à-vis* treatment of individual patients or the special training needs of junior professional staff.

Many might ask why such a purpose statement is needed as everyone knows why the health service, a hospital or paramedical department exists. Such an assumption is not well founded in that depending on who is asked and in what context, a myriad of answers could be given. A private hospital might be in business primarily to care for patients or primarily to maximize profits – which of the two is superior will determine its structure and its policies. A public hospital needs to decide, for example, whether its prime purpose is health promotion, illness treatment, care, research or teaching, or whether financial limits represent its main aim. The primacy of purpose needs to be thought out, accepted by all directly involved, and used as the guiding structural, developmental and training light.

Job design is an integral part of organizational design or development and has been discussed in Chapter 3. The principles behind designing a structure within which jobs are placed also needs some consideration. Health organizations are often large and almost always complex. This complexity derives from size in part but mostly from the large numbers of different departments and support services that exist. They are interdependent and they may have different values, philosophies and aims which are not always consistent with the organization's purpose. Such differences exist especially within the professional groups.

Structural multiplicity

Clarity and simplicity are not easy to achieve. Militating against them are the facts that whatever formally-stated and published structure exists, other structures may exist as well. First, there is the apparent structure [2]. This is the one that people within or outside it perceive as existing. Differences of perception may exist because people have not been told explicitly enough what the new structure is and because they do not fully understand the new arrangements they continue along old lines or with bits of the old and bits of the new they do appreciate. Differences of perception may exist wilfully in that some do not wish to change and continue to work to the old structure or some other hybrid.

Secondly, there is the informal structure. This is where the formal structure may well be understood but there are people in it that prefer to make their way, using their own informal lines of communication and accountability which can, of course, take on the aura of conspiracy and create significant friction. Most frequently, informal structures are relatively harmless except that they often create separate communications systems and isolate useful or important individuals.

Thirdly, there is the extant organization. Despite what is published and stated, this is the one that actually exists. It may differ from the formal structure in that it is openly recognized that certain lines of accountability or communications formally stated do not work and different, more effective ones have taken their place. When this happens it is clearly time to review the formal structure and bring the two into line. The important point is that managers, in reviewing their part of the organization, need to recognize such differences and that they may create confusion, conflicts and work against each other. The aim should be to take sufficient account of the apparent, informal and extant organizations and to ensure they and the formal structure are in synchrony. In this way people will be clear about the structure and each part will support the other parts.

Structural aid to communications

In reviewing the organization of a department, the manager needs to be clear that certain very practical matters are given sufficient attention. The length of lines of communication can be critical. The basic rule is that they should be as short as possible. It is already established that messages get distorted with the best will in the world; a long line of communication encourages or even causes distortion. The well-known First World War communications gaff caused by a long communication's line was the way a request to 'send reinforcements, we are going to advance' became distorted to 'send three and fourpence, we are going to a dance'. Almost all organizations at least in formal terms are hierarchical and pyramidal in shape; the flatter the pyramid with the fewest possible levels in the hierarchy, the better the communications are felt to be. Such flatness, whilst reducing the chances for distortion, may also take out a level of management in the hierarchy [3].

In Fig. 6.1 the same number of operational staff are managed in both cases but in the 'flatter' structure the lines of communication are shorter and there are three less middle managers.

Such may bring about significant improvements in the ability to truly delegate authority to, say, the first level of management and prevent a level that may not really have a role, if delegation is genuine, trying to create one to justify its existence. The disadvantage of taking such a development too far is that too much is expected of one level or individual. Clearly, therefore, a balance needs to be struck between flatness of structure and the scale of the span of control of individual posts.

Span of control in line management

Traditional organizational theory suggests that the most effective size of group to be managed is six to eight. With fewer staff, be they managerial or basic grade, the manager of the group loses economies of scale and, unless he is a working manager he may well not be fully occupied and will try to justify an existence by interfering, not genuinely delegating and even operating outside his prescribed role. With more staff to manage, especially if supervision needs to be close the degree of

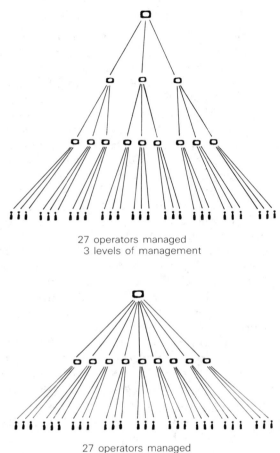

27 operators managed
3 levels of management

27 operators managed
2 levels of management

Figure 6.1 Schematic representation of a 'long' and 'flatter' organization structure. ◘ = managers/supervisors; į = operators.

management can become cursory and superficial. This means there will not be adequate support or direction, that some individuals will be treated partially and the cohesion and understanding needed in the department will be lost. This notion of the ideas span of control, as it is known, can conflict with the need for a flat structure. There is no ideal or standard model to follow, the manager needs to strike a balance and review the balance from time to time.

With the evolution of organizational design, especially those areas involving quality circles, autonomous work groups and the significant increasing use being made of external management consultants, management contracts and contracted-out services in the health services, the spans of control can be widened. Consequently, organizations can become flatter although this can be at the cost of controlling planning and work as directly or closely as in the past. As such organizations become looser in the structural sense the work to be done and the standard of quality needs to be specified and contracted for with great care. The greater need for a high commitment to vertical and horizontal communications needs to be satisfied, as in looser structures there is greater freedom assumed by the workforce as to who they go to for help, support advice and even direction [4].

THE NATURE OF AUTHORITY

A balance also needs to be struck in getting the level of responsibility of collateral managers and staff on a par and equitable. To have ward sisters or senior physiotherapists operating at ostensibly the same levels as colleagues of the same grade, particularly the same profession, but in real terms having widely divergent levels of authority and responsibility, will cause ill will amongst the individuals concerned and ambiguity in the organization or department which will create confusion. In determining the levels of authority and responsibility that should exist at each level, an understanding is needed that merely because such components are formally defined, does not mean they exist. The nature and degree of that authority need to be accepted by the individual who is going to exercise it and the level of authority needs to be accepted by the people over whom it is exercised. Normally, in the sort of cultures that exist in the health services, and more particularly the professional groups, this is not a major problem at the outset. Levels of authority can, however, become skewed over time. This can be caused by the subordinate staff losing respect for their manager for some reason and in effect withdrawing their consent to be managed in the way defined by the organization. The organizational or formal authority still exists, for it is defined in the job description and assumed by the organization charts. The personal authority – that is the authority the manager has as a result of his performance and the respect with which he is held, has been reduced. Repair work is necessary either to build the individual up in the eyes of staff, to bring the level of personal authority up to the level expected by the organization, or to formally recognize, by changing the structure through the job descriptions the reality of the situation.

In addition to authority, individuals and groups wield differing amounts of power. The authority an individual has tends to exist by virtue of the organization formally investing it in him or informally acknowledging it. Power exists as a result of specific qualities such as being a representative of a group or having some element such as money or resources which can be used at the will of the individual or group i.e. he or it has control by virtue of some extraneous element. Such phenomena must be recognized especially in and between different professional groups (see Chapter 7).

The important point to remember is that things do not happen just because a structure has been redesigned and job descriptions re-written. They need to be made to happen through people and the qualities they have personally, using the structure as a framework to support them and to make sure staff know who is expected to exercise specified levels of authority and responsibility.

Complicating features – committees, secondary organizations and conflicting values

If managers are being held to a more personal form of accountability, this will put the role of committees and other subsidiary functions in perspective. Arnold Weinstock, when appointed as head of General Electric Company in the late 1960s, sent out a directive that all committees were to be disbanded and that managers were to be held personally to account for achieving their objectives. For too long it had been possible for managers to push problems to another level of the organization, or more frequently to a committee. Such action implied the committee would be responsible and also result in decisions, when they emerged at all, being very late. He then went on to say that he had no objection to managers setting up new committees or advisory groups, as long as it was clearly understood that the managers were responsible for achievement and committees could not be blamed and were able to help the management process, not to obfuscate it. The characteristics of committees and working groups are well known by most health managers and whilst they have their uses and considerable benefit in a multiprofessional organization, especially when used with economy, in reviewing a management structure they must be seen as of secondary importance.

In addition to the danger of being diverted by subsidiary groups such as internal committees the role and status of truly secondary organizations need to be considered. The most notable secondary organizations are trade unions, and professional organizations. Significant though they are, they depend for their existence on a primary organization such as an employer or industry like the health service. Organizationally there are two points of note. The first is that secondary organizations usually exist to fulfil representative functions, (another example is the Community Health Councils). Where a representative group exists, there is an expectation that it will be consulted about change or even may want to promote change. Such a function has a degree of legitimacy, the degree will depend on the issue and the culture of the respective organizations, so any change in a management structure may need to be discussed with a professional organization or trade union, particularly if members' interests are involved. The second point is that secondary organizations would not normally expect the primary organization to structure itself in a way that is in accord with the secondary organization's structure. A trade union, however, would see it as quite natural to adjust its own structure to make it consistent with a reorganization of the primary organization, so that it could do its own work better. This happened in 1974 with health service unions and to a lesser extent in 1982. These two points serve to indicate that managers need not take account of such organization structures although they would be advised to consult with them over matters of employee or professional interest. It is then for them to adjust their structure to run in synchrony with the primary group.

Recognizing the different values, aspirations and dynamics that exist in most departments, but especially ones in which members of a profession work is crucial. Such differences are natural but if they are not recognized, and to some extent incorporated into the design of a structure, the potentials for conflict and friction are considerable. It will be of no practical use to imagine they do not exist. Healthy and constructive comment and criticism is useful and even conflict can bring about a much clearer and accepted purpose or process. The manager of a professional group needs to concentrate on areas of common interest and build on those so that by osmosis the professional elements become fused, or at least consistent with the aims and purpose of the department. In turn the department's organization and activity promote the aims of the profession and the aspirations of its members, so that there is an understood interdependence, not, as sometimes occurs, an antipathy between them or as is sometimes the case an antipathy between two professions. Conflicts of these sorts were generated during the NHS restructuring following the Griffiths Report of 1983 [5]. In a number of employing authorities it was only after very lengthy consultation that many new management structures were implemented and only after they had run for some time that interprofessional conflicts and friction between managements and professional groups began to be reconciled and settle down.

As a manager makes changes to a structure it needs to be published so that there is a clear understanding of what it now looks like. In doing so obsolete parts must be rigorously discarded so that organizational stratification is avoided, which only serves to confuse. Then, although the process of evaluation and review should be regular, a period of stability is needed so that all concerned can get used to the new arrangements and make them work.

STAFF DEVELOPMENT AND TRAINING

Having redesigned or revamped the organizational structure so that it will help the active pursuit of the department's aims, the most significant developmental activity can now begin. This is the development and training of the people within it. The terms development and training are used to describe the process of equipping those who do a job, to do it effectively, to prepare them for future work and to some extent to prepare them for future career moves. In the health services there has been considerable ambivalence about the status and commitment given to training. Some forms such as basic professional training and some postgraduate training are well resourced in terms of time, money and facilities. Other forms, like job training for some staff groups and more especially management training, have up to the latter half of the 1980s been regarded as having a very low priority.

Training as an investment

A key question any manager must ask, and answer, is why train? It costs money, often takes people away from their job, sometimes makes people dissatisfied with their job, in that it gives them ideas which may not be possible to implement, and equips people to leave for a better job. In any case, received wisdom indicates that it cannot be afforded anyway because the money is better spent in other ways such as direct patient care. Such reasons and disadvantages do not really ring true. There is a strong belief, often manifest in mission and policy statements, in and outside the health industries that investment in training is worthwhile. Training is more and more being seen as an investment [6], on which the return should be, amongst other things improvements in both quantity and quality of work done, and a way of harnessing the energy of staff.

Responsibility for training

Management training or development is no different from any other form of education or training, as far as the process is concerned. Because it is a relatively new feature to many, it is often seen as different from what is regarded as skills or job training. The subjects, knowledge and skills may differ but the principles, as well as the process, are all similar. The mystique often surrounding various training activities needs to be dispelled. Training is the responsibility of the line manager and is to do with the development of appropriate skills and know-ledge in people. Specialist trainers have a major role to play as advisers, helpers, supporters and designers – in short they are staff officers or consultants who provide a support service to the line. It will be helpful to outline the process through which training needs can be identified and satisfied. The model de-scribed is germane to many forms of training but has been developed with management training most in mind.

Management training has considerable breadth and includes any influence or experience that helps to improve managerial effectiveness. This infers that every day-to-day activity gives the potential opportunity for a training experience, if looked at closely enough and used as well as continuing to make use of formal courses and other organized training events. Training can be seen as cyclical; it is a continuous process of reviewing and doing, so that over a period there should not be high peaks or deep troughs of activity. It also helps to weave training into the fundamental fabric of the manager's job. A systematic approach gives the manager a framework and even a timetable to work to which brings some degree of order to the process and its outcomes.

Identifying overall training needs by setting objectives

The start point is clarity of role and purpose. When discussing the development of an individual this implies significant reliance on the job description either in its traditional format or as an outline of how the job is seen at the time. Within the context of the job description and knowing what the department's or organization's priorities are for the coming period – usually but not necessarily a year – it is possible to discuss and agree objective targets or priorities for the coming period. Objective setting is almost a subject in itself and the technique of manage-ment by objectives was developed in the 1960s. This process, described by John Humble [7], encouraged managers to set ob-jectives for a department within the policies and constraints of the organization and from these distil a manageable number of key results that the individual manager must achieve. Progress would be reviewed regularly and any barriers getting in the way of progress coped with. Any changes in direction, objectives or key result areas would be built into the process. The important thing about objectives or key result areas (which are the areas of management activity that must be performed to a given standard by a given time to enable progress to be made towards an objective) is that they must be quantifiable, achievable in a given time, precise, challenging but realistic and there must not be so many of them to cause problems in achieving any or all of them. Objectives need also to support and help reach the overall aim or purpose of the department; if it does not they will be diversionary at best and destructive at worst.

An objective of improving the outpatient services is virtually meaningless. Phrased in a definitive way it takes on much more relevance, for example 'to increase the number of outpatient attendances by 5% within six months with no additional revenue consequences'. Such an objective is clear, finite, quantifiable, hopefully achievable and, of great importance, it is possible to know if it has been achieved in six months' time.

Different types of objectives

There are a number of different types of objective, some of which are to do with maintenance. These are concerned with keeping levels of service, quality and cost within current limits or to aim to improve standards in existing services without changing the mix of services. Such maintenance is not just a matter of jogging along – very often it takes a great deal of effort and time because circumstances, such as recruitment, staff turnover, relationships, may change and have an adverse effect on current work. It is always, therefore, important never to forget the maintenance aspect of a work plan; it should be seen as the core part of the job that then forms the springboard for the innovative sort of objective.

Innovative objectives are those that involve taking initiatives or changing the patterns of work substantially. In health service terms examples would be to shift the emphasis from institutional to community-based work, to identify new areas for efficiency or to respond to new and different demands placed on a department by changes in technology, or the pattern of disease. The tendency is to consider innovative objectives as the most important. They may be the most interesting and they may represent a more visible target and measure of sucess when achieved. They can therefore be somewhat seductive and can siphon off disproportionate amounts of time and money. It is because of these dangers that the importance of maintenance is emphasized and the usefulness of planning so that all types of objectives can be set together and an ordered programme evolved.

The third type of objective is concerned with people. People need to be developed but if investment in this is to be effective such development needs to be planned. Individual managers and staff need to have both performance plans, which outline the targets they need to reach to be judged as performing to an agreed standard, and personal development plans which are to do with their own training and improvement. Such plans may form objectives in themselves but more commonly should form part of, and contribute to, the overall aims and objectives.

Such objectives are likely to be long term and large enough to need breaking down into their component parts and then fixing shorter periods for achieving these subobjectives. Care must be taken to ensure that the order of the component parts are sensibly and logically arranged so that achieving the first promotes achievement of the second and so on. Others will be short term and achievable within a few weeks or months, in which case, subject to maintenance, new objectives can be considered.

Negotiating objectives

The setting of aims and objectives needs to be a joint exercise in order to iron out practical snags, attain clarity of purpose and commitment, for it is largely the achievement of these for which a manager will be held to account. It is hardly practical or fair to hold someone to account for something that he did not agree to in the first instance. It is also clear that performance improves with the level of commitment to an objective or aim so practical considerations are as important as ethical or quasi-moral ones.

One of the processes that needs to be incorporated with objective setting is the setting of standards. Basically standards have two components, quantity and quality. Recent developments in the field of quality promotion are addressed in Chapter

7. It is mainly for the manager to decide what quantity of work needs to be done, to what standard or quality, in discussion with the staff involved. The engineering and electronics industries more than any other, but food and retailing as well in the last five years, have come to regard quality as important as quantity. Standards in one are not possible to set or achieve without standards in the other.

It is when the manager is setting objectives, more than at any other time, that he needs to stand back and view the whole of his responsibility. Seeing the wood for the trees is the old expression to define this process and the ability to look at the whole field of responsibilities, mainly from above, but to some extent from all angles, is much needed in managers, if they are to get all the component parts of their department into a cohesive order and the aims and objectives of all their staff meshing in with each other. Most managers in the health professions feel guilty or uneasy about standing back from their department to have a good overall look at and to think through its design and objectives but this is part of the managerial job. The ability to look at managerial issues from above as if one is in a helicopter and view the whole problem and not merely its component parts is one of the attributes that distinguishes very effective managers from the merely good [8].

DETERMINING SPECIFIC TRAINING NEEDS

There is little use in agreeing objectives for a subordinate manager, however correctly the process has been done and however many of the right criteria have been met, if there are barriers that get in the way of achieving them. The process of recognizing, defining, and analysing these barriers is one of the key joint tasks in the whole process of developing managers in their job. Some barriers, on analysis, are apparent rather then real or can be got round with relatively little effort. Others, often to do with resources or policies (some of which may be outside local control) hardened attitudes or levels of training, skill or knowledge, will need addressing. Such barriers must not be trivialized or denigrated by suggestions that 'they can be played by ear', or that 'it will be all right on the night'; if they exist they need to be dealt with. In so doing other barriers may well be made less formidable as well as pushing progress towards objectives. The overcoming of barriers may form a substantial part of a manager's key result areas or work plan but unless done objectives are unlikely to be met.

It follows that there must be a joint understanding by manager and subordinate as to which barriers are key and what plans are needed to overcome them. This joint process helps to build a relationship between the two which not only amounts to a form of contract but also ensures that the process is a continuous and organic one involving reviews of both objectives and training needs. If the process is to determine objectives and identify training and other needs for achieving them and be a development and training experience itself, it must not be allowed to become mechanistic, wearisome or a process to be gone through merely because it is policy. If the objectives and barriers are imposed or identified by one level of management and then merely passed down the line without joint commitment, the process will become mechanical and fall into disrepair. Imposition should not be disguised by diluted consultation. Jointness means joint and full understanding and agreement which infers a form of negotiated contact between two levels of management. Both manager and subordinate now should have a clear, precise and measurable definition of what is aimed to be in the coming period. What remains to be done before the cycle is complete is to identify the gaps in knowledge or skill the individual has, fill those gaps, get on with the work and then review performance and in so doing start the next cycle (Fig. 6.2).

With clear aims the identification of training needs is itself an integral and indispensable part of the whole process. The one potentially difficult part of the job of identifying training needs is that it is a process of highlighting features that might be seen as weaknesses. This especially is the case when dealing with professional groups and may appear threatening or make individuals apprehensive and so they may become withdrawn or uncooperative. The process needs to be seen as part of the overall business of management and is concerned with filling gaps and supporting and equipping people to do better. If the process is genuinely developmental, with training needs being tied into organized objectives and, to some extent, career

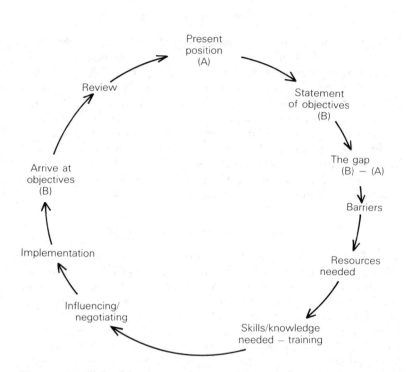

Figure 6.2 The objective setting, training and reviewing cyclical contract.

aspirations, it loses any threatening ambiance and takes on the aura of challenge and opportunity.

Satisfying training needs

In some ways the identification and satisfaction of training needs can be looked at as a bargain or quid pro quo along the lines of 'if I accept the objectives will you as my manager ensure that I have the skills to achieve them?' The more explicit the training needs are the more practicable it is to satisfy them. Some, however, especially those concerned with the general management of personnel, are difficult to be precise about. In such circumstances it may be a lack of confidence that is being identified and for this there can be a number of cures – coaching, attendance at training events, counselling and jointly looking at the performance and level of skill of managers who are recognized as effective. One of the most effective ways of increasing confidence is to encourage a member of staff who has a problem to give some thought to it, get the answer 70 or 80% right and then take a deep breath and implement it in the knowledge that the manager will give support whatever the outcome. In other words promote the notion of risk-taking where the attitude in this instance is to have a will to succeed but a willingness to fail on occasion. The important element is to agree what the gaps and training needs are and to set out an explicit programme for their satisfaction.

Different forms of training

The nature and forms of training are legion and a knowledge of them helps a great deal in formulating constructive plans and programmes for individuals and groups whose members have similar training needs. Most natural is the manager teaching an individual to do a particular thing for the first time or showing them how it can be done better. A development from this is for the manager to get someone who has the required skill or knowledge to show or inform the learner. Such a method has in the past been referred to as learning by 'sitting by Nellie'. In its worst form a learner is sat down by someone who may or may not be motivated to teach. The required skills may be learned but also many bad, out of date or even irrelevant processes too. Bad 'sitting by Nellie' training only comprises the learner watching the teacher do the job and then after a while going off and doing it for himself. However, in its best form such training, whether done by the manager direct or by an expert colleague, can be very effective. The tenet of 'tell, show, do' needs to be followed. First, the learner is told what is to be done, why and how. All three are important so the task itself can be understood and the reason for it and how it fits in and contributes to the overall scheme of things. Secondly, showing the learner how to do the task in steps if the task can be split up into component parts. Some tasks will need to be shown a number of times, some only once, but there will soon come a time for the third stage – that of the learners doing it themselves. This should be under supervision with comment made on parts that are not done to a defined standard or in the way shown. The learner should do it until he has a confidence in himself. The work he then does on his own can be checked so that unwanted or inefficient elements can be smoothed out or excluded if they should have crept in.

An extension of this method of training, especially in management skills, often involves coaching on the job. Coaching is a continuous process between manager and subordinate; its very continuity recognizes the fact that training needs to be taking place all the time to cope with new events, issues or techniques, as well as the need for individuals to be kept challenged by having their potential realized progressively. A number of managers do not coach very well. Some because they do not see it as their responsibility to train subordinate staff, some because they feel they do not have time or at least rationalize that this is so, some because they lack confidence. Most people who coach at one time or another find they lack confidence to coach because they think their coaching implies some criticism of the subordinate staff which may easily be misunderstood. The way confident coaches overcome this is by making the process one that is seen as helpful and gives learners new skills or knowledge that they can feel are of use to themselves as well as the organization. It follows that coaching is best done by managers whose overall management style is participative or involving. Where the style is less democratic the expectation is that managers plan, direct and control and the consequence is that decisions or processes are expected to be implemented fairly inflexibly – often to the letter rather than the spirit. Such a style prevents subordinate staff using their inventiveness. Learning from experience is an important part of management coaching as long as the manager is there to support the subordinate and help use the experience in a learning way. Coaching in a participative way is a continuous process and one in which both manager and subordinate recognize that both can learn from it and the subordinate especially must be allowed to practise what is being learned. Analysis conducted on managers who are recognized as being good at coaching [9] showed that the most important qualities they had were:

- they were interested in people and their subordinates particularly.
- they needed to know the potential of their staff and their aspirations.
- they searched for this potential and looked for ways to stretch subordinate staff.
- they were people-orientated and a coaching manifestation of this would be that they would develop a subordinate to deal with issues rather than take them on board themselves. It follows that coaches need to be good delegators and so,
- they needed to have and show they had confidence in their subordinate staff and wanted them to succeed.

Coaching, in addition to satisfying the tenet of telling, showing and doing, makes provision for the individual's initiative and inventiveness. It involves encouraging a subordinate to want to develop into the present job and in the longer term to equip him for furthering his career.

Knowledge, awareness and some skills can be imparted by listening and reading. Managers of professional staff seem somewhat variable in the amount of keeping up to date with new techniques or ideas they achieve by these relatively simple methods. In some professions there is an expectation that one's manager, the profession or the organization at large ought to shoulder the burden of keeping every professional and manager within the health professions well informed. Whilst such bodies undoubtedly have some responsibility in this field, the prime duty rests with the individual. Books, research papers, journals representing one's own as well as other professions, symposia and conferences all fall into this category but those involving reading, rather than listening, tend to be least enthusiastically used.

By far the most visible and concrete form of training is the course. The term covers a multitude of training or development events, ranging from the half-day seminar or workshop on a specific topic to a long (sometimes several months) development programme held away from work, often in an academic institution such as a business school or management college. Courses can be designed and organized by the manager of a professional department as is the increasing trend in some professions or for long or specialist events, internal experts or external bodies should be commissioned to do the organizing and design work.

Such groups will also have prearranged, off-the-peg training events available, which, used with discretion, have a number of advantages – most notably their relatively low cost. Whenever an individual goes on a course, his manager should invariably have decided with him that it fulfils a specified need and that it is a high priority. The manager should also always discuss with the course participant what support will be given when he returns and what it is that is expected to be learned. At the end of any course there should be a further discussion to check whether the course aims were achieved as well as to give the individual support and confidence to implement use and practise what he has learned. Too often experience shows that people are sent on courses as routine because their name has come to the top of a list, sometimes as a reward or even to get them out of the way for a while.

Often course participants come back enthusiastic to try new ideas out or do things in a different way. At this point, unless the manager is truly supportive, the department and the manager who, in the meantime have not been away but have been getting on with the routines of working life, will often not allow such innovation either actively or through inertia or indifference. The result is that frustration is built up to the extent that it may have been better for the individual not to have gone on the course at all. The ideal combination is to integrate the qualities learned off the job with the duties and tasks required of the individual on a day-to-day basis. The training then becomes central to the job being done and central, therefore, to the whole management process.

There are so many courses available and the way many are advertised and marketed makes managers feel they will be letting their staff down and become out of date if they do not participate in most of them. Many are very worthwhile but many are run with more emphasis on making money than training appropriately. When deciding on a particular course give thought to the quality of the course organizers [10]. Will they tailor the event to some extent to the needs of the individuals attending the course? Are the trainers, instructors or lecturers capable, up to date and do they have relevant experience?

Is the syllabus itself relevant to the identified training needs? Are the methods of teaching and learning up to date and appropriate to the subjects and participants? Is the course material of an acceptably high standard? The length of the course should be geared to the subjects being learned and the depth to which they will be learned. Courses should not be padded out to fill, say, a week when three days would do the job effectively. Participants being away from work cost money and usually the longer the course the more the organizers charge. There is, however, little point in nominating someone for a course that is so short that the manager feels no confidence that the training needs will be satisfied. Overall the better the employing organization knows the training establishment and vice versa, the more appropriate and effective the training is likely to be. The working arrangements, philosophy and style of the employing organization are understood but this should not preclude investigating new course organizers. Even if they are not then used the process will sharpen up existing providers of training, including those who organize it from within house.

Job rotation and time out

It may well be that for an individual the best form of training is to do a particular job for a while. Acting up, rotation, and developmental transfers are examples of this, or particular facets can be developed by giving the individual a project to complete. Such methods all give genuine experience to the individual and as long as training needs are properly identified and training procedures, whatever they are, fairly applied, suggestions of patronage or singling privileged people out will not occur. It is quite possible to have a published policy on such matters and almost invariably where this is the case allegations of partiality are few. More frequently the process is seen as helpful to the organization and useful to the individuals involved. Further advantages of such schemes are that there is the chance to see how someone copes with or grows into a job and as such it is a useful promotion or recruitment indicator. Most importantly, it gives the individual the chance to have a go at the job in the confidence that failure will not necessarily be seen in the same light as it would in a substantive post.

The crucial elements in deciding what sort of training is right will depend on the training need, the ability of the manager, organization or external training establishments to provide the right training at the right time, the commitment of the individual, availability of cash and whether the person can be spared for the duration of the training if it is off the job. The important point about all forms of training or development activities, particularly for professional staff who have job and professional aspirations, is that training should not be seen as a once and for all process but a dynamic continuum and be viewed as an investment which has a rate of return.

REVIEWING PERFORMANCE

The development and training model now only lacks two stages. The first of these needs no discussion and that is the fact that the skills learned need to be used to make sure they are practised and work is done in a more skilled, competent and productive way.

The second is the process of reviewing or checking that what has taken place so far is on course and to make sure that future objectives and training are in line with the organization's needs. Most organizations review their overall progress and performance. Companies submit annual reports to shareholders and most hospitals submit to annual reviews by health authorities which in turn report to regional health authorities and the Secretary of State. Such has always been the case both generally on overall performance and specifically on *ad hoc* issues. What has not been so common is the comprehensive review of performance, aims, objectives and training needs, of individuals within a hospital. In the past, if someone did well, they may have been given a pat on the back or if badly they may have been counselled or disciplined, although this was rarer. In any event the standards by which their performance was judged were often somewhat nebulous if they existed at all. More recently, with costs and efficiency being scrutinized more closely, with performance indicators being applied throughout the organization and with professional standards being developed to a higher and more detailed degree and, most of all and with emphasis being placed on personal accountability, greater stress is being given to individual performance review. More and more this is being seen as a formal requirement partly because some senior managers' pay will depend upon it, but more universally to ensure that a comprehensive and constructive form of performance review takes place on a regular and cyclical basis.

Appraisal, staff reporting, performance review and staff development programmes are some of the names given to the process. Each system has its own nuance, some are primarily designed as merit award tools, through which staff are, or are not, paid bonuses or awarded salary increases and there may be little emphasis on training. Others, like most of those in the health services, try to concentrate on objectives, future performance and the training and development needed in the individual to perform.

The main feature of a system whose purpose is mainly to concentrate on future performance and the training needed for it, follows quite closely the contents of this chapter. An important prerequisite is the frame of mind both parties have before any form of review is conducted. There should be the attitude within which review of appraisal is a natural part of management, that it is a useful tool for agreeing objectives and training needs and that although a formal appraisal using forms and structured discussion may take place say once a year, the process itself is a continuous one. The need for such continuity is that objectives and circumstances change as one training need is satisfied and another emerges. The naturalness of the process is enhanced by regular and confident use. The virtue of a once a year (more or less frequently depending upon circumstances but at least regular) formal appraisal is that it sets a time at which both manager and subordinate take time to review the past year, set objectives for the next period and agree training needs, having identified good and bad qualities, or at least strengths and weaknesses in the person being appraised.

On a national basis, nursing staff have had an appraisal system for ten years but it has fallen into some disuse because it is still seen as a chore separate from normal management activity and is done only in formal session. 'Done' is the appropriate word for the process for many hospitals. For the manager it is a job that has to be got over with and for the appraisee it is a process that they have to be put through. Such attitudes are common mainly because appraisal is seen as a one-off annual, or two-yearly, event with little or no review of performance on an informal basis in the meantime.

The criteria for success are similar to the rest of management activity. The process review must help make the individual clear what is to be done over the coming period and what the barriers are, clear how past performance is regarded and clear as to what training needs exist and that these will be met in a scheduled and committed way. By and large the paramedical and nursing professions now see these as positive criteria that can best be met by routine informal appraisal or review of work and regular, normally annual, formal review. The formality of the annual appraisal and the paperwork needed to make it effective have put managers and subordinates off the process in the past, as has the feeling that the process is being imposed by a higher level of authority so it does not feel owned by those that use it. The paperwork, however, is merely a tool to assist in the process. It helps get some system and commonality into the minds of both parties; it provides a check list; its very presence helps to distil thought and make the process more analytical and objective and it forms a record for the two parties. Performance reviews lose their value if used for purposes other than review and training (such as references or even in extreme cases discipline) because the confidentiality and intimacy and integrity that are needed for the process are then lost.

The preparation for a formal appraisal takes time. The manager needs to make sure that a meeting is fixed well in advance between himself and the appraisee so that both can give thought to it. This time will give the appraisee the opportunity to think about how he has performed, what changes might be made to the job and its objectives, what barriers and problems have cropped up that need to be dealt with, what his personal aims are and what development he needs for all of these. The manager goes through a similar process. Then at the appraisal or review meeting all of these subjects are discussed in detail in a joint and confidential setting. It is in this process that the paperwork becomes important and useful for not only does it help to give a systematic framework, it creates a record for the next major review in a year's time and for intermediate reviews if they are needed. The paperwork needed can take a number of forms. There are many appraisal systems published and it is a relatively easy matter to design a bespoke one for a department or hospital or to adapt or use an existing one. The most recent system designed by the National Health Services Training Authority [11] is designed as a framework which can be adapted in the context of local circumstances. Because of the significance of appraisal and performance review, a system adopted for non-pay related review from the National Health Service Training Authority individual performance review system is included in Appendix 1.

The process of performance review is a reflection of the whole process of job design, setting objectives, deciding training needs and as such is a formal manifestation of the cyclical contract outlined earlier in this chapter. What then needs to take place are regular less formal checks on progress with support being built in when needed. In addition to this, the whole system needs to be seen as a motivational one in that as well as clarifying roles and objectives it is one in which the individual can be told how well, or not, he is performing. In motivational terms no-one works well if they are treated in an indifferent way. Two phrases commonly heard are 'If only I was clear what needs to be done and what the priorities are' and 'My manager never tells me how I'm doing'. Whether or not such complaints are justified the cyclical system and appraisal systems outlined here will help make sure such criticisms do not get voiced in future.

REFERENCES

1. Handy, C. B. (1976) *Understanding Organisations*, Penguin, Harmondsworth.
2. Pugh, D. S., Hickson D. J. and Hinings, C. R. (1971) *Writers on Organisation*, Penguin, Harmondsworth; Newman, A. D. and Rowbottom, R. W. (1968) *Organization Analysis*, A Guide to the Better Understanding of the Structural Problems of Organizations, Heinemann, London.
3. Child, J. (1986). *Organisations – A Guide to Problems and Practice*, 2nd edn, Harper & Row, London.
4. Smith, M., Beck, J., Cooper, C. L. *et al.* (1982) *Introducing Organisational Behaviour*, Macmillan, Basingstoke.

5. *NHS Management Enquiry*. Letter to Secretary of State for Social Services from R. Griffiths (leader of enquiry) 1983. (Griffiths Report).

6. National Health Service Training Authority (1986) *Better Management, Better Health*, NHSTA, Bristol.

7. Humble, J. (1970) *Management by Objectives in Action*, McGraw-Hill, London.

9. Riegell, J. W. (1952) *Executive Development*. A survey of experience in fifty American corporations, University of Michigan Press, Michigan.

10. Taylor, N. (1966) *Selecting and Training the Training Officer*, Institute of Personnel Management, London.

11. DHSS (1986) *Individual Performance Review*, Circular PM(86)10, DHSS, London.

Chapter 7

Managerial and professional conflicts

Whilst this chapter is about the conflicts that can crop up between general management and some of the professional groups and between one profession and another, its main concerns are the conflicts and human relations problems that a manager of any group of health professionals will face from time to time. It addresses conflicts that occur within the organization as it is structured as well as those which occur when reviewing the sorts of organizational design which were discussed in Chapter 6. From that chapter it is clear that people at work in health-providing organizations operate in a very complex environment. They also have personal and professional values and principles, attitudes, moods and behaviours which are superimposed on this complex environment so it is to be expected that conflicts occur from time to time. It is how such conflicts are handled that often determines how successful an organization is.

If they are handled quickly and constructively, conflict can be a positive force. If, however, they are managed in a desultory way or even ignored in the hope that they will go away, they can escalate to the point at which they become all consuming of time and energy as well as destructive in their own right. Some analysis of the discord that can occur between a general management and a profession and between two or more professions has already been made.

The most visible forms of such conflict occur when the status, role or position of one group is threatened or questioned by another without too much consultation and involvement from an early stage. There is also a tendency amongst many professions to hold that the only group that can legitimately change what a profession does is that profession itself [1] and if this right is put under threat conflict results out of which, if badly handled, will create friction and tension to a destructive degree. The better situation is where a profession is sensitive to the demands placed upon it, can criticize itself and as a result keep its organization and functions in tune with external demands placed upon it. If it cannot do this in an overall organization as complex as a health service, it must be expected that external influences, such as government, will be brought to bear and either reorganize around a professional group which may isolate it, or force the profession to change.

THE PROBLEMS OF STRUCTURAL CHANGE

Problems facing professional groups

Particular vulnerability is felt by any group or individual during an organization restructuring and many lessons have been learned by those who have been through major reorganizations, as in 1974, 1982 and 1984, in the health services. Reviews dealing with particular work groups such as the Briggs report [2] also create considerable apprehension often for long periods. At such times the future status of a profession is seen as being under threat. Apprehension and friction may be increased by the fact that as a result of any restructuring affecting a multi-professional setting there is a certainty that one or another group will tend to gain power, kudos or negotiating strength, at the expense of other groups. Those groups will then feel under threat and react as they see appropriate.

Examples over the past ten to fifteen years can be cited that have worked in two ways. First, in the early 1970s the nursing profession started a process, which to some extent is still continuing, whereby it aimed to relieve nurses of non-nursing duties. Whether or not that was or is a good thing is not the point. The point at issue was that such a policy was to have a profound effect on other trades and professions which in turn reacted in various ways. Many tasks, particularly domestic and clerical, were shed with little depth of discussion amongst the groups to which they were being delegated. Friction followed, which in most areas had to be dealt with by increasing staff in those groups, partly to mollify the friction. Where significant consultation and discussion took place the friction was negligible and in fact the principle of taking on what had previously been seen as nursing duties was welcomed as, taken constructively, it could be used to enhance another trade.

Secondly, there was the philosophy of extending the role of the nurse. Whereas relieving nurses of non-nursing duties was seen as having a certain logic in that there was little point in paying nurses for doing relatively unskilled and mundane tasks that can be performed by cheaper labour, unless economies of scale were lost, the extending role of the nurse was, and in some areas still is, seen as a direct threat to other professions. The reasons behind the policy are not important at this stage but the effects and the way the changes were handled are. Nurses were planning to take over some aspects of doctors' work, for example the administration of intravenous drugs. However practical and, in overall terms, desirable such developments may have been, the threat posed to the losing groups was considerable, partly because the threat was a real one but more because much of the process of implementation was unilateral. Had it been recognized that friction would be created, it would have been possible to ameliorate its effects and even turn it to joint advantage. In most places this was not done and some interprofessional antagonism still exists. Where the development was seen as joint and all affected and interested groups were involved fully, they all benefited as for all of them it created a capacity for further development, a clarity of what they were in business to do and a much clearer understanding of what the other professional groups did. Unless such understandings are striven for positively, each of the professions will only grow in a haphazard fashion.

Disagreements between medical laboratory scientific officers and medically qualified pathologists (who were joined by graduate scientists) as to which group should be in charge of the management of NHS laboratories have existed for twenty years. In 1980 such a disagreement developed into an acrimonious dispute in the Fife Area Laboratory which in turn resulted in a three-man team being appointed to inquire into the causes of the dispute and to make recommendations. That team discounted the notion of a single head of department. It decided that there should be a departmental management structure based on consensus decision making by all the professional groups involved [3]. Embodied in that recommendation is the philosophy of joint decision making and participation – the significance of which cannot be overestimated when dealing with transactions between different professional groups. Squabbles will take place over who does new work or works new techniques, all of which can be avoided by prospective and sensitive joint planning and discussion.

The professional hierarchy

The key element or guiding principle to ensure that such a constructive process takes place is for genuine, rather than a lip service, belief to be held that the patient is the prime *raison d'être*. For some groups the patient has been viewed as a convenient raw material on which to practise a profession with other professions being of a greater or lesser, but always subordinate, use. If the patient is seen as the centre of the circle or the prime mover, the roles of the medical, diagnostic and therapeutic professions all fall into place (Fig. 7.1). In most cases, although there are some big exceptions, such as some community services and services to the mentally handicapped and other groups of long-stay patients, the medical doctor and what he does for the patient is the prime reason for the patient putting himself in the hands of a health organization. The doctor also takes the major responsibility for the patient's treatment and to some extent the care.

From then on depending on the needs of the patient each of the professional groups has a particular job to do to support the patient and doctor. Lines of demarcation and even of overlap can be adjusted according to need and circumstances, rather than being based on dogma and some over-riding uni-professional idealogy.

OPERATIONAL CONFLICTS
WITHIN THE ORGANIZATION

The more common forms of differences, conflicts and friction derive from the day-to-day working of a department or organization. They are to do with the fact that individuals and groups

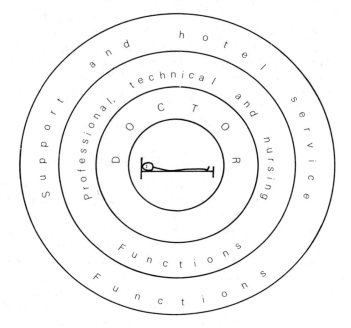

Figure 7.1 The position of the hospital patient relative to professional and support services.

do not always agree with what needs to be done and how it should be done or when. Usually the differences amongst reasonably motivated staff are small and little notice is taken of them by anyone. Often they do not get in the way of progress or the activity of a department and may stimulate thought and debate, so creating an energy that is put to constructive use. At other times, people can agree to differ. This is, however, only a sensible option where the agreement is based on respect and trust and not merely a rationalization to forestall further argument and proper resolution. Where this happens, irritation at least will be caused which may develop into the nursing of a grievance.

Recognizing differences

One of the fundamental functions of management is to get commitment from staff to certain action which involves recognizing that people have differences [4]. It must also go on to recognize that those differences can be overcome with explanation, compromise and bargaining to the extent that all involved then pull in the same direction. For such a resolution to take place there must be a clear understanding of what the disagreement is about. This applies whether it is to do with the group that is managed or only an individual. Often the point of disagreement is understood implicitly but where it is not, the manager and those involved should have it in mind to get clear on it before discussion really gets under way. It can often be the case that disagreement or conflicts arise only because both groups have different notions in mind. When this is the case an acknowledgement of it may be sufficient to bring about resolution.

Conflict of objective

It may be the objective that creates conflict. This most often occurs between a manager and a group and frequently is behind the disputes between employees and trade unions during pay negotiations. More parochial examples readily come to mind, normally where change is envisaged, such as a need to change a shift system or rosters. The conflict will be lessened if there is a clearly understood, superordinate goal such as a definitive improvement in the standard of patient care or treatment. If this is the case the parties should concentrate on this. In cases where there is not such superordinate goal, or if there is one but it is not seen as worthwhile by both sides, then the conflict will centre on the originally stated objective, in this case the shift or roster change. If there is a degree of mutual gain, perceived or real, in making a proposed change, any conflict that does exist can be put into a better perspective. Benefit that is seen as unilateral will tend to generate friction merely because of its unilateralism and the polarization of attitudes that that creates. Such a change that is seen only to benefit one side would be where financial savings were going to accrue from a shift change and not reinvested in a worthwhile project.

The wise manager will try to get as much mutuality or common interest in the objectives and aims of the department so that all participants gain materially or in terms of status. The difficulty that most managers have is that a number of other aims and issues often get tied into such negotiations. When this is the case the manager must recognize the fact, identify the differences and either set them aside with the guarantee of resolving them later or if they cannot be separated out, resolve them prospectively or as a package incorporating the main aim.

Defining the real issues

Here he should be careful not to confuse the main issue with subsidiary ones. If the aim is to save money and changing the shift pattern is the manager's way of doing it he ought to make that very clear and be willing to listen to other ways of meeting the aims. It might be that the staff group involved would be quite happy not to have locums to cover absence, or when someone leaves to cover the vacancy amongst themselves rather than have current shifts disrupted. The savings might be just as great but if the manager is adamant that shifts must change, he may well lose the ability to achieve the real aim as well as lose a great deal of goodwill into the bargain.

There may well be total agreement on an overall aim but for some reason, disagreement on how it will be achieved. Unless there are solid reasons to the contrary it may be practical, once the aim is agreed to suggest to staff, especially professionally trained staff, that subject to constraints such as safety and an ultimate deadline, they can and should decide on how a particular aim should be achieved. Such a way of avoiding conflict is not opting out, it is very much more in tune with a participative or involving style of management than the autocratic style which would demand the manager stated the aim and the method for achieving it. A great deal of work in commercial manufacturing and the public services is organized on such a participative basis. Many of the lessons learned, that have brought this about, were learned in the motor manufacturing trade with the major leap forward being made by Volvo at their plant in Kalmar in Sweden [5]. Here they evolved a system of autonomous work groups each of which had about 12–20 workers and with whom production targets and standards were agreed. From that point on the group decided who would do what, when and how. Not only did production rise to a limited extent but the amount of conflict dropped, a fact manifested by the reduced number of trade disputes. A participative style, therefore, brings two distinct benefits – improved motivation and less wasteful conflict.

Facts as a source of friction

Whilst facts should, by definition, never be in dispute, they sometimes are. Such dispute is usually caused by one group not having access to facts in the same way or at the same time as another so that it is the appreciation or understanding of them that creates a tension. Very often information is seen as power so a less than confident manager will often withhold information in whole or in part to give him such power or at least impute that he is more powerful than otherwise. Such a way of working is hardly compatible with a participative style but many still use it both parochially and in national negotiation with trade unions despite legislation that calls for disclosure of information for the purposes of collective bargaining [6]. Disagreement can also arise because the same fact is interpreted differently or because it is seen as more important by one group than another. Explanation, careful definition, clarification and sharing of information are the only practical ways through such a problem and with a modicum of patience, sensitivity and trust it is a practical process.

Conflicts of principle, value and standard

Where the disagreement or conflict is brought about by differing values or principles, it is usually at its most difficult. The values an individual or group has are those fundamental tenets that they believe in or the standards they attach to an issue. Similarly, a principle is that which guides or directs all their actions so it follows that proposals for change that either contravene or even do not actively promote such values or principles will be very difficult to bring about. For most of the time in health service employing organizations such basic clashes are rare mainly because those joining them have values and principles that are largely in accord with, or reconcilable with those of the organization. Again issues of principle arise in negotiations with trade unions, the biggest example of which in the 1980s in the

health services has been that of competitive tendering or privatization of hotel services. This was seen as a matter of major
principle by the ancillary staff trade unions which mounted
national campaigns of protest which in the event had little
impact although a degree of ill feeling remained over three years
after the process started.

At a more local level, the sort of major conflict that can arise
as a result of differing values or principles is very much in the
professional and clinical arena. The ill treatment of, and cruelty
to, patients especially (but by no means exclusively) in long-stay
areas has been relatively commonplace. Similarly, the particular
treatment of some patients by some professions is viewed by
others as ill treatment or cruelty. Within the express or implied
codes of ethics that professions have, there is a responsibility
imposed on those who see such malpractice to do something
about it. There have been a number of scandals in hospitals to
do with malpractice and cruelty, the most significant of which
was brought to a head by the nursing staff and their union (The
Confederation of Health Service Employees – COHSE) calling
for strike action in protest at its members not being listened
to concerning both malpractice and cruelty at Normansfield
Hospital in the south-west London suburbs. As is sometimes
the case with such scandals, a public committee of inquiry was
set up [6,7]. Out of the inquiry and books written [8] following
it came a recognition that differences of professional standard
might exist but where those differences are so great and one of
the extremes causes mistreatment of patients or unacceptable
pressure on one of the professional groups, there must exist a system or a process that that group, or an individual can use to make
a complaint. Such a view recognizes that if conflict is channelled
it can be managed and even some good or constructive change
may result. Preconditions are that all the parties are aware of
their professional ethics and standards and appreciate those of
other health professionals. If a complaint is made in good faith
complainants must be confident it will be seriously received and
investigated with there being a confidence that no recriminations
will follow. Most progressive employers in the health sector
have such formalized procedures.

Conflicts of principle and value exist in more prosaic form
in most professional departments from time to time. In such

departments they are normally related in part to a clinical or professional issue, hence it is important to be very clear about the issue, the nature of the conflict and the relative responsibilities of each profession. Such clarity, and recognition of how strongly a principle may be held may bring about an adjustment to the original objective or the way in which it is achieved. As long as the new objective is consistent with the overall direction of the department and contributes to the superordinate aims of the organization minor compromises are often all that are needed for resolution. Where two opposing principles are held onto implacably, damaging conflict may result before a solution is finally reached and even then there could be a residue of ill will. Managers would do well to be sure that their own values are appropriate and their principles are fundamental and not merely strongly held prejudices. Whilst discussion or negotiation are taking place there is always hope of resolution.

PREVENTING AND REDUCING CONFLICT

It may be that some competition between individual groups is healthy and productive but if the interests of those groups are in conflict or if a department is structured so that it merely makes working difficult then it is clear that structure needs adjusting. As discussed earlier, structures and organization must positively promote work rather than merely allow it to take place. Finally a clear view of the various roles of individuals and groups involved is needed if confusion is not to creep in and cause conflict where initially there was only difference. If roles and objectives are not clear their confused contribution will cause a drop in productivity or achievement and, often, tension in all concerned.

Planning to avoid resistance to change

The able manager is the one who recognizes the potential for conflict and plans to avoid it. Relatively trivial or mundane issues can escalate into full-blown disputes if not managed and handled in a timely, thorough and sensitive way. As most such issues are to do with change and much of that change is initiated by the manager, with careful planning most differences can be avoided, dealt with or even used to create constructive energy. Planning and sensitivity are the main qualities needed. When a change is initiated by the manager, he should plan in some detail how he intends to consult on the change, what are the important preconditions for success and how implementation should be dealt with. Though sensitivity is needed in this process it is especially important to be sensitive to issues that are initiated by subordinate staff groups or to be aware of the climate and feelings that exist. Such might indicate that difficulties lie ahead which if not picked up and dealt with could develop into differences, tension, conflict and then dispute. A certain amount of judgement is needed to determine what might become an issue if not addressed and what might not, but a knowledge of staff, the profession and the working climate will help in that.

Handling conflict

The nature and cause of the tension or conflict will often indicate a way of handling and resolving it. Conflict should not always be seen as negative. Its handling can be positive and the tensions created by the existence of countervailing views can be used creatively. By the very discussion about them it is possible to draw out points that might never have otherwise been thought of and which may be very useful to the department or issue in hand. Also the process of discussion and resolving the issue can be used to draw the dissenting participants together into a much more co-operative or collaborative whole.

It is possible to prevent an issue creating conflict by suppressing it. This is only a practicable proposition where individuals or groups do not feel overly strongly about it – in other words it is not a major point of principle. This can be done by isolating those who hold the counter view by getting a large measure of support for the proposition and emphasizing its moral or practical superiority, whilst denigrating the quality of the counter views. This will create a sense of rightness for the proposition which in a small work group will be difficult to oppose. Similarly, it may be possible to stress the importance of team work and that deviency from the norm will imply disloyai'y and uncooperativeness [9]. It then becomes difficult, except for strong-minded individuals or groups, to pluck up the courage to argue their case. This is an example of developing and applying group pressure which is one of the more powerful influences that can be engendered in highly skilled or professional groups. It can be, however, a two-edged sword in that if used too much, it can itself cause dissention, frustration and division, which in the medium and long terms may outweigh the short-term benefit. It may be a practical proposition to not even acknowledge the conflict or its cause. The 'I see no ships' ploy is used a great deal by politicians and managers especially when rather short of facts. In effect they are relying partly on their status and authority and partly on the fact that the people involved do not feel so strongly about the point at issue, that they would come into open conflict about it. Again, using such a ploy too frequently when the manager claims that he is operating a participative style, will bring that claim into disrepute, although on occasion it can be a very effective gambit if the manager is held in some regard.

Avoidance of conflict

Conflicts can be avoided altogether if it is possible to remove either the element causing the difference or the person or group prosecuting it. The first can be difficult in that it probably means back-tracking on an original proposal for change but a lack of conflict may be a better price to pay than forcing the issue for the time being. In any event one of the most important qualities in being able to avoid or resolve conflict and dispute is the ability to recognize that all parties to a dispute have a point of view and that there may be value in compromising. On the other hand it may be propitious to back off, do some conditioning and then try again later.

Secondly, removing the protagonists may also be difficult but it may be possible to get them to change shifts or location in order to reduce their ability to pursue their case. Such methods, again, can only be used in a most discerning way and are more difficult to employ during the run-up to a conflict than after it is resolved. In such cases these may be mechanisms best used after the event to try to prevent similar issues creating heat in future.

Confronting the issue

There will be occasions when there is little point beating about the bush. Then the best thing to do is to confront the issue by defining it very clearly for all concerned, listening to any strong views held and then deciding either what precisely will happen or to push the issue into open conflict and let the protagonists sort it out. This is a form of conflict resolution in which issues or points of difference are precipitated into conflict which some commentators [10] believe brings about quicker resolution with less subsequent ill feeling, than letting the issue drag on. A particular climate is needed for such a style and although such a method works quite well in aggressive organizations which run to very tight deadlines, such as newspaper printing and financial institutions, it is doubtful if it is a valuable method to use more than occasionally in a health setting amongst professional groups.

NEGOTIATED AGREEMENT

Almost all transactions involve a form of negotiating. From early childhood negotiation forms part of everyday life – 'will you give me your *Beano* if I let you have my *Dandy*?' – and so becomes a natural activity both at home and work. At work transactions with managers, staff, colleagues, patients and so on often have an element of negotiation in that one party wants something of the other and in order to get it a bargain involving a quid pro quo or a compromise is arrived at, often without needing to appreciate the process that is being conducted. For more serious subjects where differences or potential conflict exist, an understanding of some of the features of negotiating can be useful. Influencing and conditioning are often prerequisites of satisfactory negotiations which were dealt with in Chapter 5. Most, if not all, issues are negotiable. The time it takes to get resolution will normally depend upon the relative strength of feeling of the participants, their relative power and the issue

itself. Most managers will only get involved in large-scale negotiations fairly rarely although the basic tenets are common for
large-scale and everyday transactions or negotiations. Some of
the rituals that are regarded as *de rigueur* in the rather dramatic
negotiation, form only a minor part in day-to-day events.

Planning a negotiation

The basic assumptions that lie behind any negotiation are important. First, there are at least two parties; clearly there can be
more as during a committee meeting. Secondly, there will be a
conflict of interest, however slight this is. Thirdly, the parties
come together to discuss or negotiate the issue because they
believe they will be better off by so doing than by staying apart
and having no influence on the outcome. Fourthly, the process
of negotiation is one of informing, conditioning, making demands or proposals, evaluating these and responding and all
parties moving step by step to a compromise position which is
finally agreed. The element of compromise is crucial. Whilst it
may not be sensible to move a position unless there is a similar
response from the other side, to go into any transaction dog-
matically resolved not to move at all will rarely bring about a
long-term constructive climate and often not even a productive
short-term solution to the issue in hand. Giving and taking in a
planned or objective way are the essences of good bargaining;
without compromise one can be right – but dead.

As with be most managerial issues, the foundation of productive debate and negotiation is planning. Of most importance
is to be clear what the issue is and that all concerned are talking
about the same thing. It is also important to appreciate the
strengths of feeling that exist not only in the other party but in
oneself and to ensure that such feelings have a substantial and
logical foundation that would stand up to scrutiny. The participants, in addition to being clear on the point at issue, need to
be clear on facts and circumstances surrounding it such as the
law, regulations, professional rules and policies as well as being
sure that each party has the authority to negotiate. Further, the
parties should decide what their objectives or targets are and
what points can be conceded or compromised on and which
ones must remain unsullied.

The negotiating process itself

All negotiations are different although there are general skills and techniques available to assist. Many people have some of these through experience and some can be trained for. The significant point in a professional setting is that there are usually high levels of professional knowledge or skill which need to be recognized, respected and used, in which case the most advantageous method of negotiating is to do it in very much a joint way or regarding the process as one of equals coming together to resolve an issue. Jointness implies that as much listening as talking goes on and will naturally tend to preclude imposed solutions which intuitively most people feel do not work well in a participative climate. The danger of imposed solutions is that one party is seen to win and one to lose and such a polarization is almost bound to have ramifications for some time after the original issue is determined. Even if in reality one party has lost more than the other, it should be possible to build in some form of compensation or face saver.

In all circumstances it is as well to remember that the parties have to carry on working and doing business together which is best done in a climate of mutual respect and trust. A manager who consistently imposes solutions on unwilling or disagreeing staff will quickly lose that respect and trust. If a manager needs to get involved in wider scale negotiations or he has doubts about his knowledge or skill, he would be well advised to seek help and support, which may come in the shape of training or being involved in assisting in higher level negotiations to learn through protected or supported experience.

Disputes or conflicts that become formalized on the initiative of a trade union or professional association can be managed through negotiation. Some organizations including many health authorities have collective disputes procedures which attempt to proceduralize conflict resolution which for some groups of staff and many issues is almost impossible. Ends will normally suggest means and if a formal procedure for resolving disputes exists (especially one which allows for shifting the dispute to higher levels of the organization which means it may end up being resolved by people who have little appreciation of the issue or the surrounding nuances) the tendency is to squeeze the dispute and its resolution into a procedural mould that may not be appropriate. Individual grievances are a different matter as the voice of a single member of staff is much more difficult to hear unless there is some system. As a result of this all employing organizations recognize the value of an individual grievance procedure which also has the virtue of making all members of staff clear that they have individual rights to be heard if they have a complaint.

Once there is a set of proposals or options emerging, as a result of the negotiating process, it then becomes a relatively easy matter of deciding which one, or which set, is the most appropriate. Often with an integrative style of negotiating where there is by definition a high degree of commonality it becomes almost a process of joint choosing and where the nature of the negotiating is more distributive (that is where there is more of an element of winning and losing,) there may need to be an element of bargaining or horse trading. In both events there will need to be some degree of compromise. Once agreement is reached it is a sensible precaution to confirm the detail of the agreement; in writing if it is complex or likely to be subject to misinterpretation in the future.

Arriving at an agreement on a particular issue is the main aim of any negotiation. A secondary but important aim of a negotiation should be that relationships at the end should be more trusting and co-operative than they were before. This applies both to the one-to-one parochial negotiation, the much more formalized trade union/employer negotation and to all the levels in between. In this way many future conflicts will be avoided and those that do arise will be capable of easier resolution.

HANDLING DISCIPLINARY CONFLICTS

Handling poor performance

Performance in a professional job has quantitative and qualitative components and frequently with professional staff it is a question of judgement as to the balance struck between the two. When the level of performance falls away and drops below an acceptable standard, the manager must act. The decision as to where the acceptable standard lies is ultimately that of the manager. Performance may have dropped off because the individual is not capable of doing the level of work because he has not been trained. The solution here is clear as long as he has the potential to benefit adequately from appropriate training. Such simple scenarios are not common.

It is more usual for there to be a combination of issues each exacerbating the other. For example, there may be domestic tensions at home which put pressure on an employee who is doing complex work for which he has not been fully trained and its complexity is beginning to impose pressure on him. Such pressures may make him go on sick leave, become withdrawn and demotivated or reduce his performance because his mind is on other things. In any event the manager needs to recognize that performance has tailed off and is having an effect possibly on other staff.

The manager needs to find out the causes before deciding what further action to take. This is one of the most common situations in which counselling or joint discussion can help. Assuming the objective to be to get the member of staff back to working to standard, rather than to take punitive sanctions then the manager should discuss with the employee the fact that performance has dropped and seek the reason for this in an atmosphere that is supportive and sympathetic. In such an atmosphere there is more chance that all the germane issues will come out in which case it may be possible to do something about each of them. Pressure relieved or support given in one or more areas will help the other areas of need. For example, if the domestic problem can be eased by a short period off work or by a short-term or even permanent change of hours or working pattern, and as long as this does not adversely affect the rest of the staff or department, then it may set in train a virtuous circle that has beneficial effects at work. If the workload is accepted as being too high or the individual's skills not altogether up to coping with it, both of these factors can be dealt with. Relative or absolute workload can be adjusted by changing the staffing pattern or numbers of staff, by changing the mix of work, by actually reducing work, though this is too frequently not seen as a viable option, or by improving efficiency by changing systems, timetables or work plans. Gaps in an individual's capability can, again, be filled by appropriate training as long as the potential is there. Such measures are relatively modest but in most cases of this sort bring about the desired result. On occasion, merely talking through a problem will make someone feel better and more valued and they will then resolve the prime issues themselves.

Managing ill health and incapability

Where there is a case of ill health or incapability which clearly makes the individual unable to do a particular job in the long term a different method is called for. In cases involving significant ill health the best medical advice that is practicably available should be sought with the individual's permission. The main questions that would need answering are to do with being clear as to what the individual's illness, injury or cause of incapacity is, whether and how much the condition will improve and will it improve sufficiently to do the job to the extent required by the manager. If there is going to be an improvement there needs to be an indication as to when it will take place.

In matters of incapability the routine is similar. If an employee is presently incapable of doing a job the manager must enquire as to whether improvement is possible to the degree needed and how long it will take. If in either case satisfactory improvement can be predicted the course of action is clear – wait, support, train and, if necessary, help rehabilitate. If, however, in either case the prognosis is not adequate in either nature or degree or even in time terms then in purist legal terms the employee is incapable of doing the job and that would be a fair reason for dismissal. Managers need to adopt a rather less purist approach in the early stages especially. There may be a way of making use of the individual's abilities in a more limited way, either by reducing the level of skill, responsibility or workload in the job to the extent that it can be coped with. This may require a reduction in hours or grade or a move to another part of the department, in which cases at least the understanding of other staff, if not their agreement, is helpful. If such a change is not practicable, it may be possible, in collaboration with other departments and external agencies, such as personnel departments, training agencies or disablement resettlement officers, to find appropriate alternative work for the individual. In large organizations the opportunities and obligations to do this are much more significant than in small ones, added to which there is a cultural element in the health professions that indicates a more supportive and compassionate approach.

In any event, staff cost a great deal to train both professionally and experientially and it may be very much to the organization's economic advantage to make alternative use of the individual. If, after looking at all the options it is not possible, then dismissal will need to take place. In most capability cases involving technical ability to the job it would be necessary to use the disciplinary procedure for whilst its prime purpose is not to bring about dismissal but to get improvement, the individual must know where he stands if he does not improve.

In cases involving purely sickness or ill health, the disciplinary procedure is inappropriate. It is hardly within the realms of fairness or practicability to warn someone that if they do not get better they will be dismissed. They need to know where they stand at each point in the process of review.

Unacceptable patterns of attendance such as absenteeism every Monday and Friday (an extreme example but not unknown) with claims that it is caused by sickness, can in many instances be dealt with through disciplinary procedures. In such cases it is the pattern of attendance, commitment to the job and the conscious conduct of the individual that are under scrutiny rather than the state of health of the individual. Whether a case is dealt with on health or on conduct grounds will depend on the circumstances and in making a judgement as to which it is the manager may well need advice.

Disciplinary rules and procedures

Attention was given in Chapter 2 to policies and constraints in an organization. Individuals make up the organization and those policies and constraints govern their actions and behaviour as much as that of groups. Some policies, in the arena of personnel management, are specifically designed for individual application. They recognize that rules and procedures are essential contributors to fairness, equity and consistency. In an open or participative style of management there needs to be room for unconventiality to encourage productive dissent and initiative balanced by clear rules that show where the threshold lies between acceptable unconventiality and unacceptable deviancy.

The start point procedurally is the establishment of disciplinary rules. There will be unwritten customs, practices and conventions which are well understood, some of which have grown up internally to the department or organization, some of which have evolved in the labour market as a whole. Disciplinary rules are normally written and either stand on their own merit or can be an extension of a convention. In any event their publication should make sure that individual staff and managers are all abiding by the same standards. Generally speaking, such rules should be concise and in any event cannot cover every eventuality. They would cover such matters as timekeeping, what constituted the misconduct – or at least give examples from which logical construction could be applied to most major breaches of good practice or conduct. Examples would include the obligation to report sickness, absence, untoward incidents and accidents properly. Logic suggests such rules should be published so individuals know where they stand and the law, through the ACAS (Advisory Conciliation and Arbitration Service) code of practice on discipline handling, recommends them also. The status of such codes of practice is similar to that of the Highway Code. The code does not constitute law but its breach or adherence will be taken into account by an Industrial Tribunal when deciding a case. When such rules are broken or standards not achieved some form of remedial action is called for. It is rare, in a uniprofessional department at least, that a rule is broken to such a degree that it amounts to gross misconduct that might warrant dismissal for a first offence. More likely are the minor infringements that are no more than irritating when they crop up infrequently but become distracting and disruptive when they become more regular.

An example would be an individual who comes to work late. A few minutes late once in a while is almost acceptable and might not even call for comment. If it escalates so that it is almost a regular weekly feature that disrupts patient services and causes some adverse comment and ill feeling among other staff, then clearly the time has come to do something. It may become sensible to use the disciplinary procedure. Every employer is obliged by the ACAS code to have one and most such procedures have a number of stages which are made up of more serious warnings at each progressive stage culminating in dismissal if there is no improvement in conduct or performance. The prime purpose of the disciplinary procedure is to set up a clear mechanism that should be followed to try to bring about improvement. Dismissal is a last resort and in some ways should be regarded as a joint failure. This procedure being redemptive rather than punitive means that even before formal warnings are given, the individual should be made aware of his conduct and its effects, and counselled that he should do better, be supported in so doing where possible and know that if he does not, then at some point the threshold to formal warnings will be crossed. Once the formal procedure is embarked upon it is important in fairness and procedural terms to follow it properly. There may even be times when despite the apparent reasonableness of disciplinary action, it may be deemed unfair because by not following the procedure, the opportunity for the individual to put his case may have been prejudiced which, in turn may affect the outcome. There will be times when a procedure has not been followed properly and when disciplinary action taken has been fair. This would be when even if the procedure had been correctly followed the outcome would have been the same. It is, however, better to get into good habits and in any case a virtue of a procedure is that it maps out the order of doing things in an understood way that then enables the parties involved to concentrate on the issue rather than the process.

As well as knowing the procedure the manager needs to be clear that he has the authority to act. All immediate managers have, by definition the authority to guide and counsel their immediate subordinate staff but different procedures and employing bodies have different rules on who can administer verbal, written and final warnings and quite frequently the authority to dismiss is at least one level removed from the immediate manager. Where the authority to dismiss resides must now, by force of code of practice, be defined for every employee and that employee informed. Other than for dismissal it is still a matter of some surprise that in asking managers, especially those who manage nurses and paramedical staff, where these various authorities lie responses are often vague and equivocal.

There will be occasions when before any disciplinary hearing can take place an inquiry or investigation is needed to establish the facts. In matters of timekeeping this is not usually the case; it applies more where there are allegations of theft, assault, fraud, mismanagement in some form of general or professional misconduct. A precondition of any such inquiry is that the manager has some grounds to believe the allegations may have some substance. Secondly, there must be a full investigation into the facts and circumstances surrounding the case and thirdly the person against whom the allegation is made must be aware of them and given the chance to explain. Only once this process is complete in such cases should disciplinary action follow.

Although it may not feel like it, handling a matter of discipline is in a very real way a question of handling conflict. A member of staff has acted in a deviant or unacceptable way and the manager in the early phases is trying to negotiate a change or an improvement. The skills and techniques of negotiation are all applicable and through that process a change for the better may be reached.

Handling employees' grievances

A member of staff may be irritated or aggrieved by a proposal or action of his manager. Usually such events are rare and dealt with in the normal processes of staff management to each party's satisfaction. Experience has shown that where resolution does not thus take place an explicit and understood procedure is needed so that such a grievance is directed at where it may be best resolved. Most employing bodies' grievance procedures have a number of stages that the individual can use if he remains dissatisfied with the responses he is getting. Almost invariably the stages equate with the levels of the management structure. Each is progressively appealed to until the grievance is resolved or the individual accepts that no more can be done. Grievance procedures exist for the benefit of individual staff to be used as a safety net if they feel sufficiently aggrieved. They also exist to organize the way in which the manager at each level is required to resolve the grievance – normally within a time-scale. Sometimes explanation of a point or policy from a higher level is enough to satisfy an aggrieved individual although pro-cedures should not be used routinely to delegate problems upwards or to slough responsibility upwards. Otherwise, middle and junior managers then are by-passed often because on pre-vious occasions they themselves have encouraged it by not resolving differences or grievances as low down the organiza-tion as possible.

Resolving friction by counselling

One of the processes useful in resolving matters to do with stress, tension, differences and conflict is counselling. Many managers, however, see it as a process very much divorced from day-to-day management activity. Some forms of counselling need to be separated out and be dealt with in a very confidential way, such as certain forms of health or stress counselling or counselling to help an individual caught up in a personality clash especially with their own manager. Mostly, however, counselling should be very much integrated into the routine transactions between manager and staff. The more managers see it as a part of their job to recognize signs of difficulty, stress, difference, tension and friction and the more they appreciate what causes them the better they will be able to resolve any conflict with their staff. The value of counselling, either direc-tional or generic, is not to be denigrated, it should be enhanced and integrated into each managers' routine activity. In health organizations providing health care it is difficult to imagine managers and professional staff who do not care for each other when they should routinely be displaying caring qualities to patients. Similarly, subordinate staff need to feel confident that seeking help does not suggest that they are inadequate or incapable. All levels of staff need to know that they will, at some stage, feel the need to talk some problem or issue through and such a facility should be readily to hand when needed rather than individuals being made to wait during which period things could worsen and have an adverse effect on the work of the department as well as the individual [11].

The three main qualities needed in a manager, and in professional or specialist counsellors, are first to be very much an active listener who can interpret accurately what is being said, reflect it back and encourage expansion and elucidation. Secondly, he must be able to understand what is being said in the context of the feelings and needs of the speaker. This requires sensitivity and the ability to appreciate and understand the feelings of others as well as the pressures and constraints under which they are working. Thirdly, the manager must recognize his own limitations in counselling and be ready and able to refer the individual to a specialist if the need should arise. As in most personnel management activities, the line manager needs to be a generalist but know when and where to seek help or advice.

COSTS AND BENEFITS OF RESOLVING CONFLICTS

In the health services one of the most expensive groups of staff are the professionals both in salary terms, in what they do to patients and in the other resources they commit. Any time spent in conflict, be it negotiating on a professional issue, resolving a disciplinary or grievance issue or dealing with an ill-health problem is well spent. However, the highest costs, in both cash and opportunity, are often incurred in the causes of the conflict and the actual absence caused through stress or ill health. The fundamental management aim must, therefore, be the elimination, as far as is practicable, of the root causes of conflict. This will create more time and resource available for direct patient treatments and care and when rare conflict does arise there will be time to resolve it properly.

In handling differences and conflict the crucial element is for those involved in professional activity at work to know where they stand. Such knowledge gives rise to understanding, helps trust and confidence, encourages fairness and even-handedness and even on its own resolves conflict when it does arise.

The tale of the disputing workman may be apocryphal but makes the point in that his department is going to be subject to a productivity deal which involved changing working methods to a uniform standard, working more as a team and getting in return a bonus of 30%. His immediate manager tried to persuade him to comply without success. The arguments of the extra money fell on deaf ears. The fact was that he would let his colleagues down if he did not change working methods to which he responded because he saw no reason to change the habits of a lifetime. The benefits were expounded in great detail. A more senior manager tried to apply more scientific persuasion learned at business school and the man remained adamant. The managing director, who knew him of old was finally brought in to try and told him bluntly, with no explanatory preparation that if he did not comply to the new method he would be sacked. He smiled and said 'of course I'll do it – no-one ever explained it properly before!'

Such methods are not universally recommended. What is, however, is that the manager must know where he stands and must create a similar foundation for his own staff in the knowledge of the style, culture and needs of the department or organization. These elements will then suggest the way each issue of change can be managed without too much conflict or if conflict does arise it will ease its handling.

REFERENCES

1. Illich, I., Zola, I. K., McKnight, J. *et al.* (1977) *Disabling Professions*, Marion Boyars Ltd, London.
2. *Report of the Committee on Nursing* (1972) Chairman: Professor A. Briggs Cmnd. 5115, HMSO, London.
3. *IMLS Gazette* (1982) Correspondence – letters to the editor and to G. Smart, October.
4. Boshear, W. C. and Albreacht, K. G. (1977) *Understanding People*, University Associates, Ltd. San Diego, California.
5. Nelson, M. J. (1978) *Veering Winds of Change*, Southampton.
6. Advisory, Conciliation and Arbitration Service (1977) *Code of Practice on Disclosure of Information to Trade Unions for Collective Bargaining Purposes*, ACAS, London.
7. *Report of the Committee of Inquiry into Normansfield Hospital* (1978) Cmnd. 7357, HMSO, London.
8. Beardshaw, V. (1981) *Conscientious Objectors at Work*, Social Audit Ltd, London.

9. Walton, M. (1984) *Management and Managing*, Harper & Row, London.

10. Lawrence, P. R. and Lorsch, J. W. (1969) *Organisation and Environment: Managing Differentiation and Integration*, Irwin, Homewood, Illinois, USA.

11. Watts, A. G. (ed.) (1977) *Counselling at Work*. Standing Conference for the Advancement of Counselling, Bedford Square Press, London.

Chapter 8

Organizational support and bureaucracy

BUREAUCRACY AS PART OF HEALTH SERVICES ORGANIZATION

A constant theme in this book has been to recognize the size and complexity of most health services. To some extent these factors provide strength in that a momentum exists that assists progress, the sheer size protects the organization against political, economic and managerial vicissitudes and creates the potential for considerable flexibility in how staff are used and treated. The size, complexity and somewhat centralized organization, direction and management tend to centre on a bureaucracy which, despite some disadvantages assists by creating some sense of direction and definition of policies and constraints that enable employing authorities, the professions and individual staff to know where they stand. This sense of direction may not be universally liked or regarded as what is best for a particular set of patients or staff, and some of the policies may seem to be of little help or even get in the way of some progress, but the very fact that they exist means managers within the organization can devote more of their time to their particular job knowing the context within which they work, rather than having to spend time creating the context themselves.

Channelling initiatives

From time to time some of the structures in the National Health Service may be over centralized and the bureaucracy out of balance. It is at times like these that managers and professional groups may feel strongly about wanting to change something at their place of work. Such a change may be disallowed or frowned upon by the higher levels of the hierarchy. There are built into the system in most organizations, and in the public health services in particular, a number of routes and mechanisms that can be used to influence what is done and, in terms of the manager's day-to-day job, there are many places from within and outwith the organization from which help and advice can be sought. In the first instance how does the manager of a professional group of staff, or indeed any manager, influence the organization locally and wider? It is easier to influence those parts of the organization that are close and linked with a particular service or profession. The structural way in which this is regularly done is through the planning cycle. By putting up analytical and reasoned arguments, which may be backed up by some objective and subjective lobbying in influential quarters, plans may well get accepted and resourced which might not otherwise be the case. The practical fact of the matter is now that all public services are subject to economic restraint and the general pursuit of efficiency. It follows that if plans are not put forward in an objective and structured way not only will no additional resources be available but the current level of service and funding may well come under scrutiny too.

Using accountability as a support

Despite a stated aim to the contrary the development of general management in the public health sector has encouraged some centralization, especially from district health authority upwards. Below that level it has, however, brought some major benefits. Chief amongst these is the notion of personal accountability, the main features of which have already been discussed. An advantage of personal accountability in the arena of influencing more senior management is that who is responsible for particular matters becomes clearer. This means that in planning and resourcing terms, it becomes a much more practical proposition for one level of management to bargain with the next. If, for example, a manager is being held to personal account for providing a service, it puts him in a powerful position to specify the work that needs to be done, the support services that are required to assist and the finances needed to fund it. Only if those are available, he could argue, would he be prepared to be held to full account for full performance. As long as his arguments are soundly based it then becomes a bargained definitive contract, whereas in the past, funding of a sort was allocated to a manager who was virtually told 'do what you can with that' which gave him no leverage at all because of the passivity of his position. Planning was conducted much more on the basis of putting in a bid for more resource in the hope that something might be forthcoming. There was no great commitment on the part of the bidder, either in making the bid or implementing the development, nor on the part of the resource allocater. Now, however, the planning process puts the manager of a professionally orientated service in a very strong position, as the manager with whom he is negotiating the contract is likely to be a general manager , who will be relying on the professional for coming up with the best plan possible for a professional service. This does not give the professional *carte blanche* to wave the shroud but as long as his plans and his management objectives are in line with the overall direction of the organization and fit in with other service plans, it will be the planned output and financial input that the general manager will scrutinize, not the detail of how the work will be done. For that he will rely on the manager's professional judgement.

The personal accountability that goes with the general management philosophy also means that as far as the day-to-day operational work is concerned the professional manager is largely left alone. The discretion is left, to a significant extent, with him to decide when to call for help and from whom. Working in a clinical and professional environment brings him into contact with many other professional groups, not least of all medical staff, and because his service is patient centred, his department will normally be highly visible to the public, the press and other bodies that have influence. All of these can be used, preferably in a subtle way, to condition the decision makers on matters of concern to the manager.

The public health services are structured in such a way that encourages the practice of internal lobbying. Members of health authorities and Community Health Councils often visit hospitals and departments, as do Members of Parliament and others. The main reason for such visits is to find out what is going on, what the problems are and how improvements can be made. Such visits present major opportunities for lobbying and influencing. Medical staff are without doubt the most influential and powerful single group in a health organization. They also have formal systems designed to channel this power and influence outside the management hierarchy and it would be naïve not to recognize and use this.

Different medical specialties have their own representative committees which send a delegate to a medical executive or advisory committee, which advises the health authority or its general manager direct on matters of medical policy or practice and on matters which it thinks will affect such policies or practice. As such, it can be one of the most powerful mechanisms and although many other professional groups have their own advisory or representative machinery, they all use, to a greater or lesser extent, the medical lobby. The drawbacks of lobbying are that it tends to encourage a view that a group cannot really have a strong argument if it is relying on a third party to prosecute it, a disadvantage that is normally outweighed by the power of the lobbied group. More important is the fact that a body that is lobbied, puts its own interpretation and bias on a case it takes up, which means that unless constant liaison takes place, the original case and arguments may get lost or at best misrepresented.

The influence of lobbying is hard to overemphasize. Political lobbying in the USA has been a significant feature since the Second World War. Parliamentary lobbying in the UK has until recently been somewhat amateurish and gentlemanly. In the last five years, however, it has become a much more cut and thrust as well as professional business. Many organizations now have paid parliamentary advisers – lobbyists – whose job it is to lobby influential members of parliament. So important is this form of influence that, now, a number of professional organizations in the health industry have appointed their own lobbyists.

Supportive power intrinsic in the job

A manager of a professional group has two other significant devices available. The first is the fact that as the manager of a department he is its leader. As such he not only has to make it clear to the group what has to be done and control the group in doing it, but he has to help the group achieve its aims. This fact gives him a certain amount of organizational power, along the same lines as being personally accountable invests power and influence in him. As the leader of the group one of his most important functions [1] is to speak for the group. This means he must understand the objectives, feelings and needs of the work group and, of paramount significance, articulate them in the group and externally. He is, in effect, acting almost as a representative of the group, as well as quantifying his own managerial needs, in that he may say to his own management that unless certain resources are allocated (say), he cannot be held to account and neither can his staff work effectively or in some circumstances at all. Having the strength of a professional department behind a manager gives him a significant amount of both managerial and representational power [2].

Secondly, a significant amount of influence and power resides in the manager of a professional group of staff because of that very professionalism. The way in which the health professions are regarded by all levels of organization and outside it, for example by the public, gives the group considerable power. The fact that each professional group makes a unique contribution through qualities and attributes gives the leader of the group both a high level of responsibility and power. He should not feel abashed at discharging the first properly and using the second as a means of improving services through influencing plans, getting constraining policies or procedures changed or by getting additional resources.

The degree to which a manager uses any of these or other mechanisms is for him to judge. They are, however, all used by different groups, from time to time, to influence or condition those who make decisions at local level in particular. Beyond the local level influence is much more diffuse. Unless a manager is also a national leading light in a particular profession, the most influence or pressure that he will be able to exert will normally be through his own profession which in most instances has a hierarchical organization focusing at national level on the national pay and conditions negotiating machinery, national working parties or lobbying activities in parliament, Councils for Professions Allied to Medicine and so on. By the time the voice of an average individual professional is heard at this level it is very faint, even if it is heard at all.

Managers of health services generally and specific clinical or professional groups in particular have in the past tended to believe that influencing and lobbying is a rather grubby activity. As a result of this, much of the public relations material and links with pressure groups is reactionary rather than proactive and so much of a manager's time spent on such activities, is used to defend past actions. When a more proactive approach is adopted to emphasize progress and explain future intentions, a more constructive dialogue is developed with the media and other pressure groups, which in turn develops a rather more virtuous circle of influencing and conditioning. It also gives a manager a feeling that he is more in control than hitherto and is having to be less defensive, factors which can considerably affect the morale of the staff in his department.

SUPPORT SYSTEMS CLOSE TO HAND

The manager works in not only a complex and large organization but one in which there are a number of systems designed to give him support. Hence, he needs to influence and enlist the support of other parts of the organization to do things and make decisions which are to the benefit of his profession or department.

Few people would expect to do their own conveyancing if they were buying a house, or to self-diagnose illnesses; they would rather go to specialists to get help and advice. Similarly any medium- to large-sized organization usually finds a need to create support systems and services within its structure for managers. A balance, usually an economic one, needs to be struck between how expert in all fields a line manager is expected to be, how much assistance comes from elsewhere in the organization and how much should come from outside the structure from, for example, management consultants. Whatever the balance, however, the manager remains responsible for the management of his department and staff and so is the one who ultimately determines how much help he wants and gets from outside his own department.

In matters of personnel and human resource management, the manager has two main directions to go in. The first should be his own line manager. The reason for this is that being a more senior manager with overall line responsibility and one who would normally be more experienced in personnel management issues, the more junior manager can expect to get not only some direction but also some coaching in the particular matter under debate and management support for the course of action he ends up taking. In any event, such discussions would be easy to initiate as the more senior manager and his subordinate would meet on a regular formal or informal basis which in itself makes the process a natural one.

The personnel specialist

The second main direction the manager can take for help in any aspect of staff management is to the personnel department or personnel specialist. The functions and abilities of personnel departments vary considerably both within and outside the health and public sectors. Almost invariably they are staff, as opposed to line, functions and as such should depend on their competence for their continuing existence.

Most personnel departments have three main spheres of activity. First, they should be able to give expert or specialist advice on all matters to do with human resource management to all levels in the organization. Hence at senior levels they will advise on the need for, content and implications of policies and at all levels should be capable of advising managers on interpretation and applicability of policies, procedures, regulations and labour law. Personnel specialists must be able to advise on the availability of techniques that are management aids and because personnel practitioners have the privilege of being able to move and work throughout the organization, can advise on morale, the state of labour relations on particular problems they may perceive.

To a limited extent they can provide advice to individual staff. Usually this should be limited to advising on procedural matters, in that if an individual was complaining about a manager the most that the personnel specialist should do is to explain how to pursue a complaint and outline the policies and constraints that surround the subject under question. At times a personnel specialist may act in a counselling capacity but usually this would be at the request of the line manager or on a matter that was non-contentious such as career guidance.

Some personnel departments provide a much more employee-orientated service than is outlined here. This is usually the case when the personnel function has developed through providing a welfare service or where trade union activity has been very low or in some cases because the culture of the organization has required it. Such a development is neither right nor wrong. Where it does not get in the way of providing effective support to managers it can be of considerable help. To do both jobs well, however, usually needs significant resources and in the health services there is not the capacity to do both well. If it is accepted that the line manager is in a big way his own personnel manager, other than when specialist knowledge or skill is needed, then it follows that he should be the person staff look to in most work-related ways including welfare. It is the manager who needs to call on expert help and he must be able to be given it with no compromise when he needs it. In short, a personnel department is predominantly a management service to help managers do their whole job better.

Secondly, a personnel specialist can provide practical help and support to a line manager. Most often this is in the shape of assisting in interviewing for recruitment or disciplinary purposes, in fact some organizations insist on a personnel manager or officer being present for all senior staff interviews or serious disciplinary hearings. He may also provide help by taking part in negotiations with staff groups or trade union representatives. In all such circumstances he is helping and to some extent advising but must stop short before encroaching into the line manager's responsibility for making decisions.

The third sphere of activity is that of personnel administration. This can be a very wide and deep activity but is essentially to do with setting up support systems to help managers manage in a more informed way, an example being computerized personnel records and information system, and doing administrative work for or on behalf of managers, such as running an advertising and recruitment service centrally because the economies of scale and nature of the work make that the most effective way of dealing with it.

The subjects in which a manager can expect a personnel

specialist to be expert, knowledgeable or skilled, in any of these three spheres can vary and have been outlined in many publications [3]. However, no personnel practitioner could be supportive to line management unless he were able to operate competently in a number of areas.

First, in the area of human resource planning and provisioning which sounds somewhat pretentious but is descriptive of a range of activities and expertises that must be available to a manager from a personnel specialist. The main components are planning, for which the personnel specialist must be able to build up an effective records and information system, organizational analysis and design, job design, job evaluation, recruitment and selection, knowledge of and ability to interpret terms and conditions of employment, employment policies and labour law.

Secondly, he must be able to assist the line manager in the field of monitoring individual and group performance, motivational theories and techniques, analysing and helping with problems such as high turnover, absenteeism, sickness, overtime and those to do with skill mixes which are either out of balance or overly expensive.

Thirdly, he must help in the development and training activities which involves the identification of all training and development needs and being able to design and run, or be able to find, events that will satisfy these needs. Part of these functions will be the development of appraisal and review systems.

Fourthly, the line manager can expect help in employee relations issues, employee services which will include the provision of staff services, such as occupational health, accommodation and social club facilities. Also expertise must exist in matters of health, safety and accident prevention, negotiating with trade unions and professional associations, the development of effective communication systems, application of policies, the law and good practice to any employee relations issue such as disciplinary and grievance problems, disputes handling and the management of issues to do with sickness or ill health. A specialist should also be competent in judging levels of morale and the state of employee relations in departments and across the organization as a whole. A skill in general counselling and an ability to refer problems to specialists is essential.

In all of these areas the personnel specialist should be able to advise and support the line manager and where appropriate set up systems and administer these and other administrative work that is central to personnel management. He will also be aware of developments in the function and changes in staff management practice and techniques and so enable line managers to keep up to date in the field.

Financial support

Depending on the way in which management support services are structured, it is likely that some financial services, such as payroll administration, will be of considerable help to managers. It is taken for granted in most organizations that the compiling of pay for individuals is done by a central department using computers although this may change in the future. These two factors mean that staff in a payroll department acquire a great deal of specialist knowledge on pay, conditions and terms of service, including knowledge of superannuation, pensions and sick-pay schemes, which is all available to line managers. In addition a great deal of personnel information now comes from payrolls so it is possible, especially through computerized systems, to get hold of information about individuals and groups of staff that can then be used to assist in their planning, organization, control and general management. It is through such systems that specialists can help managers make the important link between staff numbers and the way they are deployed and financial budgets and performance against these. There are two caveats however. The first is to do with confidentiality. The Data Protection Act, which came into force in 1986, regulates the use of personnel data held in electronic systems and users or owners of computers that hold any personal information must register with the registrar. He will only grant registration if he is content that all the regulations governing the sorts of information held, why and how it is to be used and confidentiality safeguards are satisfactorily met. The law at present does not cover hard copy or information held in paper and manual systems but most employing authorities will have a policy that sets the same standard for both electronic and hard copy. The second is that whenever a manager is reviewing the department structure or making changes in work patterns, he will need to assemble the cost implications of such changes more and more accurately as pressure is exerted to make managers more accountable in budgetary terms. Such precision is often only possible with expert help and normally that would be available within a finance department.

Work study and organization and methods support

When examining the structure, the way work is organized, the levels of performance, skill mixes, work flows and the physical layout of a department there will be, in most large organizations, a management services department, a work study team, or research team that will be able to give advice and conduct surveys or analyses of particular blocks of work or organizational structure. The names such departments have, have different shades of meaning but most are available in a department, usually called a management services department or management support unit. It will be composed of trained staff who are specialists in the various subjects cited, who on request will conduct a study or analysis and submit a report and recommendations to the manager.

Like the personnel department, a management services department is a support or staff function – it cannot make decisions in its own right – it can only advise and help line managers. Usually, however, if its advice is sound the manager will take it into significant account but always he must remember he will be responsible for his own decisions and he may have to take other matters into account when making them. In the public health services the bulk of management services departments' time has up to recently been taken up with working on incentive bonus schemes for ancillary staff groups. With the demise of many such schemes their time has been freed up so their capacity to assist in wider aspects of management is considerably greater. Their major expertise lies in being able to analyse the organization of work in departments and making recommendations on improving efficiency, which will enable savings to be made or more work to be done using the same resources without overloading them.

The virtue in sometimes using such a body, or even employing external management consultants is that apart from their technical expertise they bring an outsider's eye to bear on any problems. Recommendations can also often seem more accept-able coming from outside the department and, therefore, easier to implement, which is why many companies use management consultants. In this way unpalatable solutions can be imple-mented without local mnagement appearing to be tainted and thus the team spirit maintained. Care as to how often such a ploy is used needs to be exercised as otherwise the manager becomes seen as ineffectual and bypassed and the department organized and even managed in some ways by outsiders.

There are, of course, many other individuals and groups, both inside the organization and outside, who can be called upon to help or to whom managers can direct subordinate staff. Examples are pressure groups, counsellors, manage-ment consultants and institutes of higher education. The degree of help or advice the manager will need will depend on the issue and his own level of knowledge, skill and confidence. Often it can be quite valid to get advice merely to confirm a course of action but doing so gives an added confidence that can make not only a difference in making the decision in the first instance but also in the manner in which it is implemented. It is important to recognize that there are a large number of sources of help, support, advice, influence and power that a manager can ex-ploit. He, however, must make the staff management decisions and be responsible for them so he should only seek enough advice or help that enables him to take action with confidence.

Professional bodies

The profession itself or professional association is often available to give advice and even active help on some matters of manage-ment within a professional group. Most significant is the work some of the professions do in the fields of human resource planning, education and training. Some, such as the College of Radiographers, already run uni-professional management courses, often in conjunction with local further education in-stitutes. The pharmacy and physiotherapy professions are also actively planning such programmes. Although such uni-profes-sional training may be somewhat parochial, in that it reduces the opportunities for cross-fertilization and can tend to promote the interests of the profession at the expense of the primary organization, it does develop managers in the context of the professional group they manage.

Self-help

One of the greatest sources of strength, however, is self-development. As well as using all the agencies available, reading, research, critical self-analysis and contemplation are major sources. They are also under the very direct and personal control of the individual manager and can be exercised at any time and are very cheap. They demonstrate a willingness by the individual to take his role and development seriously, which is of benefit to the organization and profession and also to the individual in his current job and future career.

REFERENCES

1. Coleman, J. C. (1969) *Psychology and Effective Behaviour*, Scott, Foresman, Blenview, Illinois, USA.
2. Handy, C. B. (1976) *Understanding Organisations*, Penguin, Harmondsworth.
3. Fraser, J. M. (1971) *Introduction to Personnel Management*, Nelson, London.

Part Four

Issues for the Future

Chapter 9

Set fair for the future?

This chapter is not intended to be the prophesies of a soothsayer but more some predictions of likely developments in the next five to ten years in matters that have an impact on the management of health professionals. It is presented to help ensure that the focus of personnel management in nursing and paramedical services in health care is on the future, recognizing that present standards and activities must be the baseline from which to start. Most of what will happen over the next ten years will be extensions or developments of what has occurred in the past. Change in most things is a continuum and an evolution of what already exists, rather than the sudden arrival of totally novel elements. This means that though some change, and, therefore, adaption to it, will be rapid, it will for the most part be evolutionary.

THE CHANGING SHAPE OF HEALTH SERVICES

This book started with the notion that management of any group of staff has to take place in the context of the workplace, wider world of the labour market, the community at large, and the economic, social and political fabric of the country as a whole. Changes in these areas have as much impact on a professional working in a hospital department as a change in clinical practice within the particular profession does.

Political constraints

In the political and economic climate, likely to pertain for some time, competitiveness, the pursuit of efficiency and economy and the philosophy of accountability are undoubtedly going to be major features in industry, commerce, public services and particularly the health services. The effects of this, as it has started to evolve, are already being felt by managers in the health work but there is little doubt that it is going to pick up momentum partly for partisan and idealogical political reasons but equally because of the shift from the public to private sector for the provision of increasing amounts of health care. Most significantly, however, although spending in real terms has increased reasonably steadily (if slowly) in the public health sector (NHS), the demands continue to outstrip supply. Over a ten-year period central funding will begin to fall away significantly as a prime source of government revenue – North Sea oil – dries up and public spending commitments remain high in other areas, such as social security and services, education and defence. The development of a frame of mind and a culture that is economy and efficiency based is no bad thing. The more efficient a service is the more work it can do. The management philosophy of personal accountability, initiated with some success as a result of the Griffiths recommendations, has laid the foundations for a much leaner and potentially effective health service. Clearly many other areas of activity will be needed to realize this potential. The tendency to over-centralize will need to be reversed, delegation should be made much more real in substantial matters rather than merely apparent. Adequate mechanisms for predicting demand for services, fair ways of rationing services, effective ways of redeploying resources to more needful areas all need to be developed. On a more organic plane, recognizing that medical professional hegemony still exists [1], to either consciously build future management structures round that fact, more than is currently the case, or develop a much more genuine and jointly participative management confederacy.

Future organizational change

In January 1989 the Government published the white paper [1a] which will bring about significant organizational change at hospital and health authority levels. Most significantly for health professionals it will force the greater participation of doctors in management of hospitals and give greater freedom to local hospitals to determine not only how they manage staff but also what they pay them. As market and commercial pressures are imposed on hospitals the overall management ethos will also change. As this evolves it is probable that as different professional staff develop and gain expertise managerially, more general managers will be drawn from their ranks which over time will not only improve career prospects for them but improve the degree of inter-professional integration, especially in the processes of staff management. The view the professions take of such a development will be crucial as they could at one end of the spectrum grasp such opportunities eagerly to the benefit of all or at the other end might pursue policies of uni-professional aggrandisement or seek total autonomy and independence which may enhance the power base of the particular profession but will not help integration and will cause significant friction on the way. Having said this, however, it is of significance, for the improvement of all standards, that each of the professions allied to medicine develop their unique bodies of knowledge, skills, ethics and the numbers within the profession so that adequate supplies of well-trained staff are available to the health services.

Moves towards commercialization

The shifts in economic fortune may have other implications on health services as a whole but the NHS particularly. With medium- and long-term effective reductions in central funding, other than general searches for economy and efficiency, two themes will evolve. The first will be charging patients for more services than is currently the case, for example for catering services and certain non-urgent or broadly defined cosmetic procedures. Such a development will not affect the staff management significantly. What will, however, is the second development which would be to develop privatization by putting out to commercial contract more services than is presently so. Examples will be medical records, computing services, personnel and other management support services and more significantly, direct patient care diagnostic services such as pathology and radiology, both of which already make some use of the private sector resources. Over the next ten years more radical changes can be envisaged which would involve the selling off of commercially viable services to the private health care sector, for which services patients would need to be insured. Such services might include certain general, orthopaedic and gynaecological, surgery, acute medical work, psychiatry related to stress, cardiac and thoracic medicine and surgery; in other words, many of the acute specialties, leaving the public sector to provide for the growing and changing demands of the elderly, long stay, community and services for children. The effects of such change on the health professions, especially in education and training matters, could be very significant and whilst such changes would be progressive, their impact particularly on training, morale, career progression and employee relations in what remained in the public domain would be significant.

There is significant debate currently taking place about internal markets and the notion of Self governing hospitals. The first of these might bring about the situation where one hospital with special expertize and capacity would charge other hospitals for them and so effective organizations might generate income.

A self governing hospital would be a hospital or group of hospitals managed largely independently of NHS control but would depend very largely, if not totally, on referrals from General Practitioners who would have freedom to refer to whichever Self governing hospitals would give their patients the best overall deal. As revenue would be attached directly to each referral only the more effective hospitals would flourish in addition to a great deal more power devolving to family doctors.

Demands for, and supply of, health care

The changing patterns of care and rapidly shifting demands, especially in community services and care of the elderly, are already showing signs of affecting the various professions, in terms of the nature of the work to be done and the amount of it, which will have a big impact on training and education, as well as the calibre of people entering the professions. Where demand begins to outstrip supply, in other words, when there is no further room for redeployment or efficiency savings, health professionals will be faced with the need for a more overt form of rationing. Forms of rationing occur now through the management of waiting lists and the way work programmes are designed to cope with the illest end of the patient spectrum but with demand and real need rising, in some areas by 4–5% a year (for example in the elderly along the south coast of England), a rationing or allocating system will be needed. Whether such rationing will be based on criteria imposed from the centre or developed locally by multi-professional groups, and whether the criteria are based on pure economics, quality of life or clinical need as determined by one professional group or another remains to be seen. Already, health economists, especially those at York University [2], are trying to devise objective ways of balancing relative needs with relative benefits and costs. Cost benefit analysis is not a new technique. Its application, however, in determining which patients get what services is to many professionals a new feature. Where demand outstrips supply some mechanism for apportioning care, will be needed more and more. Only if all professional groups are involved in the design of such mechanisms will managers of professional staff and the staff themselves be committed to the outcomes. The absence of such a commitment will create a great deal of confusion and friction as well as inter-professional contention.

Legal limitations

Professional groups need to be aware that development in the legal field, mainly in respect of litigation, will accelerate. In the USA most people providing and receiving health care are very litigation conscious and very large sums for damages are now commonplace and the sheer number of suits is high. Commentators protest that developments to the same extent are just not possible in the UK. This may be so but over the past twenty years, triggered partly by the thalidomide episode and more recently (1987) by awards of damages of hundreds of thousands of pounds and in one case of over one million pounds, the health care consuming public has become much more aware that it has rights and remedies when negligence of any sort by any care group is involved. Such awareness has brought about a slight reduction in the mystique that surrounds most health care professions and in the main they have started to respond constructively. Significantly the principle of fully informed consent is being adopted by most of the professional groups especially medical professionals in certain specialties. Such a development, however, takes time and patience. It, and the increased propensity to sue in cases of negligence, means that the standard of total care needs to be raised, systems of recording have to be meticulous and open to scrutiny. There could develop an increased apprehension on the part of health professions to practise any but the most conservative forms of health care and treatment unless a system of 'no fault' compensation is introduced. Each of the professions has, in turn, stated that it does not wish to practise with a lawyer on its shoulder and whilst this is partly in the hands of the courts, the health professions can be influential by raising their standards.

CHANGES IN THE LABOUR MARKET

A political and social theme that has been quite visible in the past few years is the need for a workforce to have a greater stake in its organization. Workers shareholdings have been encouraged as have co-operatives and partnerships. Some commercial organizations have even negotiated reduced pay rises in return for rights of share ownership. Such a development poses problems for the public service and health services especially. The trend in the NHS is to make it more accountable to the consumer and the community that it serves and in so doing emphasizing that the ownership of it rests with the community. On the face of it such a trend is inconsistent with employee shareholding, except in the moral sense. In this respect it is possible to motivate staff through emphasizing that they hold the health services in trust or stewardship for the community at large, which stresses their importance almost to the point of indispensability. Many commercial companies try to engender a similar ethos, claiming that staff are their most valuable asset and the quality of product as well as quantity depends almost exclusively on them. The difference is that there is a material reward and commitment with such a commercial shareholding which does not exist in the public sector. For managers to pursue the concept of shareholding in the public health services too far will bring it into conflict with the public ownership notion.

Involvement of staff in the way they do their work and in contributing to policy formulation – in short, participation or a form of industrial democracy, are much more practicable developments to concentrate on in the NHS, and to varying degrees already take place. Such systems of management only satisfy certain needs in employees, however, and the limitations as well as the benefits described in Chapter 4 need to be considered.

New technology and skill polarization

Changes in the economy, system of work, clinical practice and technology have over a period polarized the workforce and the labour market. At one end of the spectrum very high levels of skill are needed so high ability or potential is looked for, which means that standards of recruitment and training have had to be raised.

Perhaps the biggest change that many workers have had to face recently is the dramatic and rapid change in technology and the use of electronics in almost every aspect of work. Robotics, computing in most aspects of life, new diagnostic and therapeutic tools that do things better and very much faster, all help to do more work to a higher standard. Such innovations, however, put strain on groups and individuals and often machines can be seen to be dictating the pace at which people work. The attitude is becoming engendered in health work that affected industrial process in the past whereby it is the machine and technology that is in control of the person not the other way round. Far from plateauing out, the rate of change and innovation is likely to increase in the next decade so the problems of changing skill mixes, changing roles and merely coping with new technology in a technical sense, let alone in the organic and social senses, will become increasingly difficult especially for existing staff. For new and younger staff who have been educated and brought up to expect such rapid change, the problems will not be so intense but different abilities and attitudes within organizations created purely by such differences in age and attitude will create further areas for tension. The manager is the one who must become an expert in the management of change and resolving differences and, better still, being able to predict them before they become manifest and plan to avoid or absorb them.

The even more rapid advances in information technology are of especial significance to managers. In the past most managers of professional staff have complained that they could manage staff much more effectively if only they had adequate information on budgets, expenditure, workload, overtime and sickness. The current state of information technology gives them such a capability and most organizations are in the process of designing information systems that will turn that capability into a practical and very comprehensive reality. The advantages, especially in the field of managing staff, are obvious. The short-term problems, however, are that some managers have rationalized their inability to manage on the lack of information and when they have it they may still not be able to cope. With their inadequacies shown up they will need careful handling and development and probably much patience. More commonplace, however, will be the training and practice managers need in handling the new information, the information they generate and how to interpret, analyse and put it to practical use. The need to identify training needs will become paramount to ensure that technical training is appropriate and also to reap the main benefits through changing attitudes of managers and staff to information and other technology so that it is seen as a useful tool and aid – not as a system getting in the way, something merely to be coped with, or even worse, controlling the professional group.

At the more mundane end of the spectrum, changes in technology have reduced substantially the need for middle-range skills, except as a training ground for the higher levels. This tends to push those people with middle-range abilities down to the unskilled and more routine end of the spectrum [3].

There are a number of personnel management implications

of this phenomenon which are most marked in professional groups. One is that moderately able people begin to find the skills they have are needed less and often the only way to remain employed is to accept that they need to work below their potential in more routine and mundane work. In addition to turning the originally unskilled people out of work, there is the danger of those left doing it becoming bored and fractious. Such is a recipe for very difficult management and also planning for long-term education, training and staffing becomes fraught. Examples of these trends are discernible in most health professions. In nursing there is a long-term policy to discontinue the use of enrolled nurses which will cut out a considerable part of the middle of the skills spectrum. At the same time the nursing profession has tried to improve its standards through increasing the entry qualifications – something every health care profession has done in the last ten years. This has two results. The first is that there are and will continue to be problems and contention about how middle-range work gets done, especially if learner nurses are designated supernumerary, and the second is that by raising educational entry qualifications, a large supply of potentially good applicants will have been cut off. This, linked with the fact of perceived low pay and that most of the profession is female dominated (thus reducing the potential catchment of recruits by half), has given the nursing profession a phenomenal planning problem, as exemplified in the Project 2000 Report [4]. Whilst the biggest group numerically is nursing, each of the health professions is going through very similar trends, the results of which the managers in those groups will be the first to experience.

It follows that managers in those professions should be trying to influence the direction in which their professions are going. Although other groups have the right to suggest what work a profession should do and to what standard it should be done, the profession has the prime responsibility to keep itself relevant to need and equipped to satisfy that need.

Practical benefits of anti-discrimination

The make-up of the labour force and the dynamics within it may give some clues as to partial remedy. An analysis of the professional labour force also throws up examples of some potential tensions that could develop destructively if not managed but could be very constructive if tackled objectively. A consistent thread running through the professional groups is the lack of balance brought about by passive and active discrimination, history, conditioning and socialization. The professions are made up largely of women, predominantly white, who are generally recruited and trained young. The attrition rates during training are moderate but after training in the first few years of professional practice increase rapidly, with relatively few returning to full-time work later in life.

The untapped resource amongst men, ethnic minority groups, the disabled and older women especially is substantial. If it were exploited, training facilities would need to be improved and some attitudes and cultures changed but the long-term benefits for the professions and the wider health services would be considerable. Additionally a greater stability would be injected into the total workforce together with a genuinely more egalitarian working environment. This book cannot attempt to resolve all such human resource planning issues but in pointing them out it can create an awareness amongst the managers of professional staff about the issue and possible ways of starting to solve them.

NEW CONCEPTS

On balance it is the search for efficiency and economy that is likely to put its mark on the management of health professionals over the next few years. To some extent this will be a fulfilling challenge. Organizations and staff within them will find it satisfying trying, for example, to improve the quality of service and the standard of professional performance. Developments in industry such as total quality concept and total quality commitment [5] place the emphasis on meeting improved standards in quality. This is to meet rising consumer expectations as to quality and as the quality of performance and production go up, the number of faults in products and the amount of re-work, or putting faults right, drop [6]. Consequently, efficiency and real productivity go up. In a service dealing with health care, the notion of striving to constantly improve quality is intuitively a good one. In practice it can also have great benefits to output and so is likely to be viewed as a vehicle that can be put to good use in reducing unit costs, and even free up resources for alternative use.

Already considerable stress is being placed on quality assurance in the health services and within the professions themselves for these reasons. This emphasis will increase in the next few years. In so doing more and more effort will be put into creating quantifiable measures by which the measurement of quality will become more sophisticated and possibly more meaningful. Whilst most of the general pressure for such developments will come from the centre and general managers, the pitfall that is most dangerous in the health services is that a topic such as quality assurance will be regarded as a separate entity and pursued only by specialists. Quality is like personnel management in that it is the prime concern of the line manager. Unless objectives and aims to do with quality are totally integrated into normal management activity they will never be achieved and, worse, frustration and disenchantment will be created as another management fad passes into history. The role of the professions and their managers in creating objectives to do with quality and balanced measures will be crucial; they will, however, need to spend considerable time and skill in their creation and at the same time will need to be clear on the relative roles of the different health professions and standards they each work to, to make sure they are not creating or defending restrictive practices.

It is in these areas and in developing their own management skills that the different professional groups face the greatest challenge within the health industry. They will need much skill and determination in creating and maintaining a balance. Most attention, as is so often the case, will need to be given to the training, development and management of staff within each professional group as if they are kept skilled to meet real needs, the professions and the organizations they serve will go from strength to strength.

REFERENCES

1. Illich, I. (1981) *Limits to Medicine. Medical Nemesis: the Expropriation of Health*, Penguin, Harmondsworth.

1a. White Paper (1989) *Working for Patients*, HMSO, London.
2. Williams, A. (1985) Economics of coronary artery bypass grafting. *Br. Med. J.* **291**, 326–329.
3. Jenkins, C. and Sherman, B. (1979) *The Collapse of Work*, Eyre Methuen, London.
4. United Kingdom Central Council for Nursing, Midwifery and Health Visiting (1987) *Project 2000 – Counting the Cost*, UKCC, London.
5. Crosby, P. B. (1979) *Quality is Free*, McGraw-Hill, New York.
6. Peters, T. J. and Waterman, R. H. Jr (1984) *In Search of Excellence*, Harper & Row, New York.

Appendix

Review of individual performances against objectives

INDIVIDUAL PERFORMANCE REVIEW

Individual's name and initials	*Date*
Job title	
Manager's name and initials	*Location/department*
Dates of review discussion	*1 2 3 4*

(with acknowledgements to the National Health Service Training Authority)

INDIVIDUAL PERFORMANCE REVIEW (IPR)

1. The background to this way of reviewing performance, identifying training needs and setting future targets is set out in the guide (based on the NHSTA guide) that accompanies this set of papers.
2. The process is designed to be cyclical and should normally take 12 months and then be repeated.
3. The NHSTA system has been adapted to take account of local circumstances and the fact that the SGH system is not going to be used for pay or merit bonus purposes.
4. Timing – the manager is responsible for the whole process and the flow chart below outlines the order/timing:

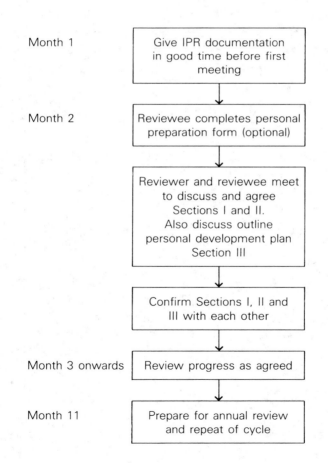

Month 1 — Give IPR documentation in good time before first meeting

Month 2 — Reviewee completes personal preparation form (optional)

Reviewer and reviewee meet to discuss and agree Sections I and II. Also discuss outline personal development plan Section III

Confirm Sections I, II and III with each other

Month 3 onwards — Review progress as agreed

Month 11 — Prepare for annual review and repeat of cycle

PERSONAL PREPARATION FORM

This form is optional but is intended to help you:
- Identify your current job and its strengths and needs   – Part A
- consider your career interests   – Part B
- express your development needs   – Part C

This is a guide to help you prepare for a useful discussion during this major review. You do not need to complete it unless you want to or adhere to it during the discussion, or show it to your manager. After the discussion you may keep this form or ask for it to be kept by the Personnel Department with you Personal Development Plan.

PART A:
Your current job and its strengths and weaknesses

(1) Which aspects of your present job give you greatest satisfaction?
(2) Are there additional skills developed elsewhere which give you satisfaction but which are not used in your job?
(3) Have you been clear what your job objectives were?
(4) In which job objectives have you done well? Why?
(5) Which job objectives have you found the most difficult? Why?
(6) Under what conditions do you work most effectively (deadlines, type of manager, working alone or with others, etc.)?
(7) What are your key job skills and areas of strength?
(8) What skills or knowledge do you feel you lack?
(9) Has your job changed significantly in the last 12 months? If so, how?

Appendix

PART B: Your career interests

(1) What is your main career interest?
(2) What are some alternative career interests?
(3) What work areas or activities do you think would lead to these?
(4) In what work do you believe your next job could possibly be in the next two to five years?

PART C: Your development needs

Look over what you have said about yourself. Now, consider what actions and commitments may be necessary on your part to pursue your work interest in the NHS. Consider primarily the next two to five years ahead.

(1) What are your main development needs?
(2) Has the lack of any skill or knowledge limited your progress in your job or career? If so, how can you overcome this limitation?
(3) What actions could be planned to meet these development needs?
(4) What additional education, training or experience do you need?
(5) Are there any other considerations you need to take into account to achieve these plans? (Mobility, personal aspects, etc.)
(6) Do you feel there are any major constraining factors outside your control?
(7) Is there any more information you need to make a realistic plan from your manager or anyone else?
Any other comments

If you would like this to be kept with your Personal Development Plan please add your name and date below.

Name .... Date ....

SECTION I PERFORMANCE PLAN

Overall **Purpose of this Job**

Columns 1–4 to be completed jointly at the start of the review cycle.
Column 5 is there in case there is a changed objective or changed timing.
Column 6 is for a review of how well objectives have been achieved. For particular aspects of performance complete
Section II.

1. Key objectives for the coming period	2. Rank order	3. Action required: who needs to do what and when for each key objective	4. Outline any personal development need. (More detail in PDP.)	5. Any changes in substance or timing of key objectives	6. Review of achievement

SECTION II ASPECTS OF PERFORMANCE AND SKILLS

This section is designed to help analyse, preferably jointly, the abilities and performance of the person being reviewed. Together with Section I and Parts A, B and C (Personal Preparation Form) it will provide the basis for the Personal Development Plan.

The appraiser should consider the appraisee's performance in each facet. (Background notes page 195).

Aspect of performance or skill	Comments
1. Organization and management of work	
2. Identification of problems and their solution	
3. Foresight and depth of thought	
4. Level and application of professional and technical skills	
5. Management and development of staff	
6. Oral and written communication	
7. Other relevant aspects, e.g. perseverance, energy, relationships with colleagues	

Overall performance   The reviewer should discuss, and here briefly record, the reviewee's overall performance.

We agree that this review and the plans in it are a fair reflection.

Individual's signature ....Date ....

Manager's signature ....Date ....

Countersignatory's signature ....Date ....
(where the reviewee requests a discussion with him/her)

SECTION III PERSONAL DEVELOPMENT PLAN

PERSONAL – CONFIDENTIAL WHEN COMPLETED

This plan should focus primarily on those learning/development needs identified in the Performance Plan and then on development needs related to the individual's realistic career expectations in the next 2–5 years. Production of the Personal Development Plan will be accepted as confirmation that a Performance Plan has been agreed. It supersedes any previous Development Plan.

Individual's name and initials	Date of completion	
Job title	Location/department	
Objective from Performance Plan	Learning/ development need	Proposed action and timing

Formal training to be specified over

Jobs for which individual could be considered – include other work areas and locations as appropriate:		
Type of position and/or function	Date (Q/Yr)	Geographic mobility

Career and Personal Development Needs:

Which work experience, special assignments, personal improvement, education and training information would be helpful to the employee?

```
┌─────────────────────────────────────────────────────┐
│                                                     │
│                                                     │
│                                                     │
└─────────────────────────────────────────────────────┘
```

Development plans:

- What have you agreed to do to meet these development needs?
- Which of you will be responsible? When will they occur?

```
┌─────────────────────────────────────────────────────┐
│                                                     │
│                                                     │
│                                                     │
└─────────────────────────────────────────────────────┘
```

Any formal training planned

Course title and subject	*Date planned (Q/Yr)*

Individual's comments

```
┌─────────────────────────────────────────────────────┐
│                                                     │
│ Individual's signature ........................Date ........................... │
├─────────────────────────────────────────────────────┤
│ Prepared by manager:                                │
│                                                     │
│ Manager's signature ........................Date ........................... │
└─────────────────────────────────────────────────────┘
```

The original of this Personal Development Plan will be held on the Personal File. One copy will be given to the individual and one copy will be passed to Personnel to help build the training and development programme.

BACKGROUND NOTES

Individual performance review (IPR): Getting the most out of the process

Why do it?
In any organization – and especially in one the size and complexity of the NHS – it is vital that managers are clear about the key objectives they are to attain, and how these relate to the work of others.
IPR is a systematic way of achieving this clarity. It also provides:

- an opportunity for the individual to know what performance is expected of him/her and to receive feedback.
- a consistent means of monitoring career needs and opportunities.
- a chance to develop a common culture and set of NHS values relating to performance and improved patient care.

IPR consists of the following activities:

- Job clarification and targetting.
  (What is my job – has it changed – what are the key objectives? What help do I need to achieve them?)
- Monitoring.
  (How are the key objectives being met – do we need to change them in the light of experience of new circumstances?)
- Review.
  (How did the last 12 months go? Use that experience to plan for the next year.)

What will make IPR work well?
IPR is a complex inter-personal process. Individual competence can be enhanced through skills training, but a great deal can be achieved simply by ensuring that:

- there are *regular* and *frequent* informal review discussions about progress, using the Performance Plan and the Personal Development Plan. IPR is *not* a 'once a year' event.
- these reviews between you are truly *open* and within clear understandings about confidentiality.
- your dialogue is *positive, supportive and forward looking* — a forum for exploring new ideas and improving performance rather than seeking alibis or excuses.
- you persevere! No Performance Review process is easy: it needs to be worked at and *will* improve with practice and feedback.

OBJECTIVE SETTING

To improve the performance of the Service we have to be clear about what is important, what should be achieved. Reaching agreement about key objectives and their proper definition is thus critical. If this is not done well, the whole of the rest of the process will contribute little to the success of the Service.

Where should objectives come from?

From your shared work experience and the organization's statement of intent contained in its Strategy and Operational Plans. These organizational objectives will have to be translated into personal responsibilities and are thus a rich source of material for Individual Performance Plans.

How many objectives should there be?

The purpose of objective setting is to ensure progress and performance on those issues which is agreed are *key* to the success of the organization. If there are too many, you will be unable to make significant progress on any of them. Do not make the mistake of including tasks that need to be done which are not key. Objectives should be sufficiently challenging to ensure progress, but achievable, to avoid frustration through failure. If your number of agreed objectives reaches double figures you will probably have too many.

How should objectives be defined and written?

Find ways of stating objectives which make them:

- quantifiable (wherever possible make them objective and thus measurable).
- capable of being tested (define the constraints within which they are to be achieved).
- within a definite timescale.
- precise (clear, well-defined and in as few words as possible).

Examples:

1. 'Improve laundry output' may not get you very far. Increase flatwork output from 20 000 pieces to 25 000 pieces per week without increasing unit costs, by 31 March ....' is beginning to give you something real to aim for. Above all else, avoid being imprecise in stating your objectives. Ask yourselves 'how will we know if this has been done?' and agree the answer.

2. You also need to be sure that you are addressing the right problem. If your objective is to reduce surgical waiting lists, you might call for improved bed occupancy in the surgical unit. But occupancy may not be the answer, you have also to think about length of stay, through-put, theatre time, etc.

What different sorts of objectives are there?

Check whether your agreed objectives include something against each of the following broad categories:

Innovation New initiatives such as securing the move to community care for priority groups; identifying areas for improved efficiency; making provision for AIDS sufferers, etc.

Maintenance Keeping up or improving existing standards of perform-ance such as maintaining financial control; ensuring continuity of essential supplies; keeping waiting time for patients in clinics with agreed limits.

Human resources To further develop the organization's human re-sources such as ensuring that your staff have their own Performance Plans and Personal Development Plans, that the investment in train-ing is realistic and linked to organizational objectives, and that talent spotting and succession planning are going on.

Whilst some objectives will necessarily deal with short-term issues, you should also be thining about longer-term goals, agreeing action that will begin to move you towards them.

How do we deal with constraints upon the individual?

To attempt to agree objectives without recognizing the constraints under which all individuals operate in an organization as complex as the NHS is a mistake and will be counter-productive. Both the objective and the action planned to achieve it will be unrealistic.

Example It would be foolish to set an objective for a manager on a Surgical Unit which called for an improvement in bed occupancy, length of stay or throughput on that Unit, without fully recognizing the part to be played by consultant surgeons and theatre staff in that change. Equally, in agreeing action needed, it would be wrong to ignore situations where your performance is dependent in part on action which can only be taken by your manager – these under-standings will need to be clarified between you.

WHO IS INVOLVED IN IPR?

Individual Performance Review is primarily a two-way process between the individual and his or her manager, supported by the Personnel Department.

1. The responsibility for the whole process and its success rests with the managers. It is their job to initiate and maintain the process for their staff and to ensure that apart from the formal stages taking place properly, informal reviews take place regularly and constructively.
2. The individual makes a major contribution not only to their own development but to the clarification and achievement of objectives that are key to the organization as a whole. They should regard the process as a 'contracting' one with their manager where both have obligations and rights.
3. The Personnel Department: in this system the Personnel Department performs two important functions. First, receiving a copy of all Personal Development Plans, they can draw together all training and development needs across the organization and initiate any new activities called for. Secondly, they can provide a 'trigger' function, both to remind managers that a major review is expected, and to keep top management informed of the extent to which Performance Plans and Personal Development Plans are current.
4. In exceptional circumstances, the individual can ask for the manager's manager to review the process. The whole process is designed to be an intimate reviewing and contracting one so the fewer people involved the more relevant the process will be. That in turn will promote confidence in it.

HOW TO USE THE IPR PAPERWORK

'Performance Review depends on dialogue, not paper!'

But despite this, paper is useful in:

- prompting a helpful sequence of thought and discussion.
- aiding consistency of approach throughout the Service.
- providing a record to avoid review and career progression.

The IPR process needs to be followed closely using the documentation as a means to an end, not as an end in itself.

Working Document (Section I)

At each major review, the manager and the individual agree on key objectives for the coming period (normally a year). These objectives are entered in Section I in Column 1. Then in:

Column 2: rank objectives relative to their importance in the achievement of overall success in the job.

Personal Preparation Form (Section III)

This form is intended to help the individual being reviewed to get the most out of the review session, by encouraging him or her to define aspects of job and career, and how these need to develop.

Use of the form is optional and it may afterwards be retained by the individual, sent for filing to the Personnel Department, or destroyed. The decision on this rests with the individual concerned.

Index